LIVING WITH

DIABETES

LIVING WITH
DIABETES

EVERYTHING YOU NEED
TO KNOW TO SAFEGUARD
YOUR HEALTH AND
TAKE CONTROL OF YOUR LIFE

Rosemarie Dainelli Perrin

Seth Braunstein, M.D., PH.D., EDITOR

ASSOCIATE PROFESSOR OF MEDICINE, DIABETES PROGRAM
UNIVERSITY OF PENNSYLVANIA SCHOOL OF MEDICINE
PHILADELPHIA, PENNSYLVANIA

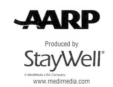

AARP

Produced by
StayWell
A MediMedia USA Company
www.medimedia.com

STERLING
New York / London
www.sterlingpublishing.com

AARP Books publishes a wide range of titles on health, personal finance, lifestyle, and other subjects to enrich the lives of older Americans. For more information, please visit www.aarp.org/books.

AARP, established in 1958, is a nonprofit organization with more than 37 million members age 50 or older. The AARP name and logo are registered trademarks of AARP, used under license to Sterling Publishing Co., Inc.

Produced by

StayWell®

A MediMedia USA Company
www.medimedia.com

Selected content and artwork have been provided by Krames Health and Safety Education, a division of StayWell, a MediMedia USA company.

LIBRARY OF CONGRESS CATALOGING-IN-PUBLICATION DATA AVAILABLE

10 9 8 7 6 5 4 3 2 1

Published by Sterling Publishing Co., Inc.
387 Park Avenue South, New York, NY 10016

© 2007 AARP

Distributed in Canada by Sterling Publishing
c/o Canadian Manda Group, 165 Dufferin Street
Toronto, Ontario, Canada M6K 3H6
Distributed in the United Kingdom by GMC Distribution Services
Castle Place, 166 High Street, Lewes, East Sussex, England BN7 1XU
Distributed in Australia by Capricorn Link (Australia) Pty. Ltd.
P.O. Box 704, Windsor, NSW 2756, Australia

Manufactured in the United States of America
All rights reserved

Sterling ISBN-13: 978-1-4027-3012-2
ISBN-10: 1-4027-3012-8

For information about custom editions, special sales, premium and corporate purchases, please contact the Sterling Special Sales Department at 800-805-5489 or specialsales@sterlingpub.com.

Contents

Biographies

Rosemarie Dainelli Perrin

Rosemarie Perrin is a science writer specializing in medicine and public health. Having grown up in a household in which her mother, sister, aunt, and uncle all had diabetes, she has a special interest in the topic. Perrin has written about diabetes and other medical and mental-health topics for print and electronic publications including *Frontline*, the CDC Foundation newsletter, and the American Cancer Society's *Primary Care Newsletter*, for which she received the Rose Kushner Award for writing achievement in the field of breast cancer. Perrin served as managing editor for two editions of the American Cancer Society's *Textbook of Clinical Oncology*, as well as an edition of the society's handbook for cancer survivors, *Informed Decisions*.

In another life, Perrin wrote about wilderness recreation: She is the author of *The Explorer's Guide to Lost and Buried Treasure* and is co-author of *The Explorer's Source Book*.

A native of New Orleans, Rosemarie Perrin now resides in Atlanta.

Seth Braunstein, M.D., Ph.D.

Seth Braunstein, M.D., Ph.D., is Associate Professor of Medicine at the University of Pennsylvania School of Medicine in Philadelphia, in the Division of Endocrinology, Diabetes, and Metabolism. He is the former Chief of the Diabetes Program at the Hospital of the University of Pennsylvania.

Dr. Braunstein received his undergraduate degree from Princeton University, graduating with Highest Honors in a combined Biology and Chemistry program.

After earning his medical degree from New York University (NYU) School of Medicine and his doctorate in molecular biology from NYU Graduate School of Arts and Sciences in the NIH-sponsored Medical Scientists Training Program, Dr. Braunstein completed an internship and residency, both in medicine, at the Hospital of the University of Pennsylvania, as well as a Fellowship in Diabetes at the University of Pennsylvania.

A principal investigator in the NIH-sponsored Diabetes Control and Complications Trial (DCCT) and the long-term follow-up of this cohort, the Epidemiology of Diabetes Interventions and Complications (EDIC), he has also participated in numerous trials funded by the pharmaceutical industry. Dr. Braunstein's current research interests include diabetic neuropathy, the prevention of diabetes, cardiovascular outcomes, diabetes in pregnancy and adolescents, and the epidemiology of diabetes interventions and complications.

A frequent regional, national, and international lecturer, Dr. Braunstein has published extensively in journals such as the *New England Journal of Medicine, American Journal of Medicine, Diabetes Care*, the *Journal of the American Medical Association*, and *Diabetes*. He has also written many abstracts and has co-authored several book chapters.

Dr. Braunstein is a member of the American Diabetes Association (ADA), the American College of Endocrinology, and the European Association for the Study of Diabetes.

CREDITS

AARP

Kelly Griffin
SENIOR PROJECT MANAGER
AARP Office of Social Impact
Washington, D.C.

Margaret Hawkins
MANAGER, HEALTH PROMOTION
AARP State & National Initiatives
Washington, D.C.

Keith Lind
STRATEGIC POLICY ADVISOR
AARP Public Policy Institute
Washington, D.C.

Cheryl Matheis
DIRECTOR, HEALTH STRATEGIES INTEGRATION
AARP Office of Social Impact
Washington, D.C.

N. Lee Rucker
STRATEGIC POLICY ADVISOR
AARP Public Policy Institute
Washington, D.C.

Illustration Credits
Some illustrations have been adapted from the original content of
KRAMES a MediMedia USA company.

Illustrations on pages 49, 50, 51, 62, 63, 65, 66, 73, 85, 86,
90, 91, 101, 105, 107, and 122 © 2006 Elliott Golden

EDITORIAL BOARD

Preface

SETH BRAUNSTEIN, M.D., PH.D.

D iabetes mellitus is a chronic condition affecting more than 21 million people in the United States and more than 190 million worldwide. If current trends continue, there will be almost a doubling in the numbers over the next 20 years, both in the U.S. and around the world. Diabetes is a condition that affects young and old, people of all races and backgrounds, men, woman, and, with increasing frequency, our children.

Diabetes is a metabolic disorder of carbohydrate (starch and sugar) metabolism diagnosed and monitored by following the abnormally elevated level of glucose or "sugar" in the blood that characterizes this disease. It also results in abnormalities of protein and fat metabolism.

Diabetes can make you feel bad when your blood sugar is too high or too low, and it can lead to long-term problems that are not easily reversible. Diabetes is the major cause of new adult vision loss, the major cause of nontraumatic amputations, and the major reason why people need dialysis or transplantation for kidney failure.

More than almost any other medical condition, diabetes requires the understanding and cooperation of the patient for therapy to be successful. A physician, nurse, or nutritionist can prescribe medication, exercise, and dietary programs, but unless the patient understands why these therapies are important—and unless the patient cooperates in the initiation and continuation of these therapies—treatment will often fail to meet its goal.

We now know from several large, well-executed studies that controlling the blood glucose makes a difference in how a person feels, and reduces the risk of the serious complications mentioned above, as well as heart disease. Other aspects of diabetes management also make a difference, such as blood-pressure control, smoking cessation, weight control, and optimal cholesterol management.

That is what this book is about—how to take care of yourself or others who have diabetes. In the chapters that follow you will find explanations and discussions related to all aspects of diabetes, from the causes of diabetes and risk factors that make people more susceptible, to current treatments with lifestyle changes and medications.

Having this information and becoming educated about this disease is really a first step in providing you with the tools necessary to take charge of the situation. You can then become an active participant, together with your health care providers, in the ultimate goal of achieving good health.

Perhaps the best way to use this book is a little at a time, picking the chapters that sound interesting to read first. The book is written in such a way that each chapter can stand alone and usually is understandable without having to digest everything that came before. Another point to remember is to reread the chapters later, picking up points that you may have missed the first time around, or that will be clearer once you have completed all of the chapters. And we encourage you to question your health care providers about your condition and therapies. The knowledge you gain in this book will help you better understand why certain procedures and treatments are necessary, and what you should expect in your care from your health care professionals.

The ultimate goal is to make you a partner in your diabetes management, which for its success requires active participation by you and perhaps help from family members and friends. This book, I believe, will help you gain that understanding.

Introduction

MARK H. BEERS, M.D.

Diabetes can be a killer, and surviving it requires knowledge, action, and vigilance. Do not neglect your diabetes, or it will destroy you. I tell you this because I have had diabetes for nearly 45 years. That makes me one of the long-term survivors. I am also a doctor and a medical writer, and I had the opportunity to review the book you are about to read. In these pages I share with you my dual perspectives: one as a person with diabetes, the other as a doctor caring for people with diabetes. What is in this book can save your life, but only if you act upon what you learn.

I have experienced diabetes as a child, adolescent, and adult. I cared for my diabetes before the advent of blood-sugar testers, when only urine testing was available. I managed my insulin before new formulations made that easier. When I was young, I boiled my glass syringes to sterilize them before disposable syringes (and long before insulin pumps) revolutionized care for people with diabetes. When I first began my medical practice, only a few oral medications were available; most were not as effective as what we can call upon today. We have tools to treat diabetes today that I had to do without for decades. They are all available to you.

Yet despite the enormous progress in diabetes care, two truths have remained constant over the past many decades: Knowledge and involvement are the keys to remaining healthy and living well with diabetes. Neglect and denial guarantee disaster.

You will learn that you cannot ignore your disease for even a moment or it will take you on a roller-coast ride of highs and lows that will leave you exhausted. Let your disease remain out of control a little longer, and you will suffer consequences that cannot be undone. You will read—and you will be told time and again—that important factors are within your ability to control. First among these is your weight. In close second place, and intimately tied to your weight, is your diet. And obviously exercise is a big part of the wellness picture, too. If you are like most people, you will not change your behavior; you will remain overweight, eat foolishly, and exercise too little. Take that approach and you will not join me in being one of the long-term survivors. It is that simple. It is that harsh.

But for all of you willing to take control of your diabetes, on the other hand, there is very good news indeed: You can avoid the complications of diabetes and lead a healthy life. Learn all you can know about your medicines, diet, and the best strategies and tactics for avoiding the complications of diabetes. But don't fool yourself into thinking that knowledge is equivalent to taking the actions required to survive this disease and stay healthy.

What you will gain from this book, and elsewhere, are tools for achieving good health, but you must use that newfound knowledge to motivate your actions, wisely and consistently. With diabetes, your doctors and other health care providers lead the way, but it is through your own actions that the battle is lost or won.

1

Diabetes Defined

If you are reading this book, there's a high likelihood that you or someone you love has diabetes. Perhaps you have a family history of diabetes that has given you firsthand knowledge of its symptoms and effects. Whatever your personal circumstances, you are motivated to learn more about the disease. And that's smart. Why?

Because, as the adage has it, knowledge is power. Informing yourself about diabetes can empower you to change your life in ways that will allow you or a loved one to live well with the disease. Indeed, you may even be able to prevent the condition's onset. So in a way, this book is all about power—the power that an individual can wield by taking control of his or her diabetes and learning how to manage it.

What Is Diabetes?

Diabetes is a disease in which the level of sugar in your blood becomes elevated over long periods of time—often years or permanently. This occurs for one or two reasons. First, your body is producing little or no insulin—a pancreatic hormone that controls how your body uses glucose and other carbohydrates. The second reason, in many cases, is that your body cannot effectively use the insulin it does manage to produce. In both scenarios, your body fails to maintain its proper blood-sugar levels.

Although the name of the disease is usually shortened to diabetes, its full medical designation is diabetes mellitus (sometimes known as sugar diabetes). In order to understand how to manage diabetes, it helps to understand a bit about the chemical reactions in your body that transform the food you eat into the energy that keeps your cells healthy and your system functioning.

Metabolism: From Food to Energy

After you eat a snack or a meal, your digestive system targets those nutrients that are easiest to convert into energy, which is really nothing more than fuel for the body. The most rapidly convertible nutrients of all are carbohydrates—a special class of organic compounds that can be changed into certain substances by fairly basic chemical reactions, including oxidation, reduction, or hydrolysis. Carbohydrates also happen to be abundant in most plants. For these reasons, they are a critical food source for animals and humans.

The vast majority of the carbohydrates you ingest are broken down by gastric juices in your stomach and intestines (and by enzymes in the body) into glucose, which is the principal circulating sugar in the blood. Blood then carries the glucose to the body's cells, most of which burn it as quickly as they can for energy. (Some cells convert the glucose into its storage form, a more complex carbohydrate called glycogen.)

To enter the body's cells and be used as energy, glucose requires an "escort"—the hormone insulin, which is manufactured in a gland near the stomach called the pancreas. Insulin travels from the pancreas through the bloodstream to the cells, where it serves as a key, "unlocking" those cells so that glucose can enter them and be used as energy. As glucose is utilized by the cells, its level in the blood falls.

It's easy to see what a crucial role insulin performs in the body. First, it manages how your body uses carbohydrates from the food you eat. Second, it stimulates cells to remove glucose from your blood. Third, it plays an indirect role in helping your body absorb and use amino acids and fatty acids, both of which are vital to the body's proper functioning.

When the pancreas is performing optimally, it senses your blood-sugar levels and starts or stops producing insulin so precisely that it keeps your blood-glucose levels within a normal, healthy range. This automated regulation system is crucial: The body's organs—notably the heart, brain, blood vessels, nerves, and kidneys—depend on normal blood-glucose levels in order to function healthily.

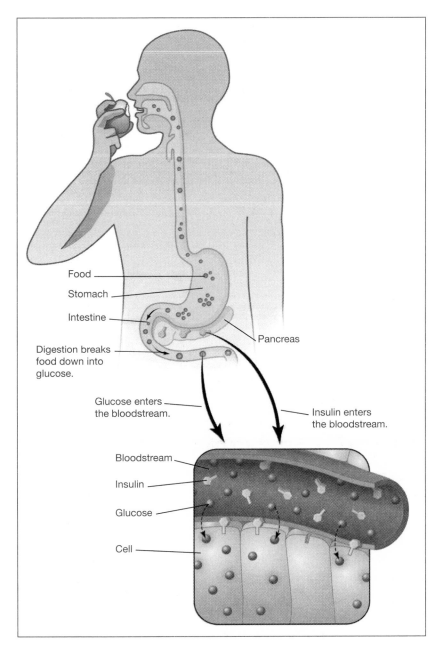

Food

Stomach

Intestine

Digestion breaks
food down into
glucose.

Pancreas

Glucose enters
the bloodstream.

Insulin enters
the bloodstream.

Bloodstream

Insulin

Glucose

Cell

> Digestion breaks food down into glucose. Insulin allows glucose to enter the cells,
  where it is burned as fuel or stored.

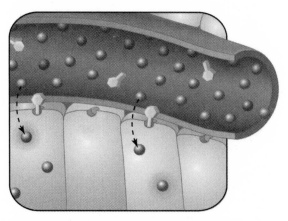

> Without insulin as its "passport," glucose cannot enter the cells.

The amount of glucose circulating in the blood is called the blood-sugar level or the blood-glucose level. This level is maintained in a normal range in healthy people. When your blood-glucose levels are checked during your annual physical exam, the health care provider will give you a number that indicates what your blood-glucose level is. (This test is usually done after you have fasted for several hours.)

When a person has diabetes, blood-glucose levels are higher than normal—above the range needed to maintain healthy tissues and organs. Over time, the elevated glucose levels, called hyperglycemia ("hyper" means "high"; "glycemia" means "blood sugar"), can damage the heart, blood vessels, kidneys, nerve endings, and eyes. A first symptom of diabetes could be related to damage in one of these body areas, but more often the first symptoms stem from the high blood glucose itself and include:

- Frequent urination, or polyuria, especially at night

- Increased thirst, or polydipsia

- Blurry vision

- Fatigue

- Lightheadedness

- Weight loss

- Yeast or vaginal infections in women

Left uncontrolled, hyperglycemia can lead to severe confusion and coma. Over time, it can cause serious health complications—including heart disease, blindness, kidney failure, and decreased blood flow to the lower limbs and nerve damage, increasing the risk of amputation.

Also, when the cells cannot get glucose to use for energy, they first burn for fuel the body's stored version of glucose—glycogen—which resides in muscle and liver cells. If they continue to be deprived of glucose or glycogen, the cells use energy supplied from fat. When the body turns fat into energy, it deposits acids called ketones in the blood and urine. A buildup of ketones (a process known as ketosis) can cause a dangerous condition called ketoacidosis. Not only are ketones toxic themselves, but they make the blood acidic as well.

The key, then, is learning to manage diabetes by maintaining your blood-glucose levels near normal to prevent both short- and long-term problems. Among the principal goals of this book is to show you how—and why—it is within your power to accomplish just that.

What Are the Types of Diabetes?

There are two main types of diabetes, type 2 and type 1. In addition, there is a third type, gestational diabetes, and a group of less common forms of diabetes.

Although type 2 and type 1 diabetes arise from different causes, they have two aspects in common. First, people with diabetes have a "genetic predisposition"—that is, an inherited tendency—to develop the disease. Second, some element in a person's environment must trigger the diabetes. Having a family history of diabetes does not mean that a person will automatically get the disease. Even in cases of identical twins, where both twins carry exactly the same genes, one may develop the disease while the other does not. Scientists are working to discover the environmental triggers that cause only certain people in a family to get the disease.

Here are the main distinguishing characteristics of the different types of diabetes:

• Type 2 diabetes is a disease in which the body initially succeeds in making some insulin, often at very high levels, but then resists its actions. Type 2 occurs most frequently in adults; indeed, it was formerly known as adult-onset diabetes. Increasingly, however, the disease is being diagnosed in young people and even in adolescents, primarily those who are overweight or obese. Because type 2 diabetes accounts for 90 to 95 percent of diagnosed cases of the disease, it is discussed before type 1 diabetes throughout this book.

• Type 1 diabetes, previously called insulin-dependent diabetes or juvenile-onset diabetes, is a disease in which the body stops making insulin. Although this type of diabetes is usually diagnosed before age 30, it can occur at any point in life. About 5 to 10 percent of all diagnosed cases of diabetes are type 1. Considerable evidence suggests that type 1 arises from a viral infection in people with a genetic predisposition to the disease.

• Gestational diabetes is a type of diabetes that only pregnant women get. It may be temporary and disappear when the pregnancy is over, but in some women it may persist afterward as well—or reappear months or years later.

• Other types of diabetes are associated with certain diseases, genetic conditions, other illnesses, or medications. These other types combined may account for as much as 5 percent of all diagnosed cases of diabetes.

Type 2 Diabetes

Type 2 diabetes is the most common type of diabetes. Not only does the pancreas produce inadequate amounts of insulin, but the cells in the body fail to use it properly. This is called insulin resistance because the cells appear to "refuse" to use insulin to convert blood-borne glucose to energy. Although the pancreas may respond by producing even more insulin, that quantity is insufficient to overcome the resistance. Over time, insulin production tends to decrease, and blood-glucose levels increase further or require more medication to be controlled.

Type 2 and type 1 diabetes affect the body in much the same way: Both prevent cells from using glucose to produce energy, thus raising blood-sugar levels. Beyond that commonality, however, type 2 differs from type 1 in three important ways:

- First, type 2 is not an autoimmune disease—that is to say, it does not result from the body's immune system attacking and killing insulin-producing cells. The pancreas continues to produce insulin, but the amount manufactured cannot meet the increased demand caused by insulin resistance.

- Second, type 2 diabetes is primarily a disease of people over 40 years old. (However, it is becoming much more common in younger adults, and even in teenagers.) In addition, ketoacidosis rarely occurs in type 2 diabetes.

- Third, whereas scientific studies have shown that diet and exercise can prevent or delay the onset of type 2 diabetes, there is no known way to forestall the occurrence of type 1. Type 2 diabetes is linked to body weight; some 90 percent of those who develop type 2 are overweight or obese. And even though the precise link between excess weight and type 2 diabetes remains unclear, it appears that fat cells—especially fat within the abdomen itself—produce substances that interfere with the production and action of insulin.

Type 2 diabetes has a more obvious genetic link than type 1—that is, it runs in families more often. For example, children of a parent with type 2 diabetes have a 1 in 7 chance of developing the disease. But when both parents have type 2, the child's risk soars to 1 in 2. By contrast, children with one parent with type 1 have only a 1 in 17 chance of getting the disease. When two parents have the disease, the child's odds of getting type 1 range from 1 in 4 to 1 in 10.

Type 1 Diabetes

Type 1 diabetes is usually diagnosed in young people, most often around the time of puberty, but it can also occur in adults and in younger children. In this condition, there is an absence of insulin. Type 1 diabetes is an autoimmune disease, meaning the body inflicts the disease on itself. For uncertain reasons, the body's immune system attacks the insulin-producing cells (called pancreatic beta cells) in its own pancreas. Some experts think that a viral infection stimulates the body to attack those insulin-producing cells.

Without insulin, cells in the body cannot absorb glucose from the blood, so the liver overproduces glucose. At the same time, however, carbohydrates in food are still being converted into glucose, and that glucose is still traveling via the bloodstream to the cells.

Rebuffed from entering the cells by the absence of its passkey, insulin, the glucose simply collects in the bloodstream. This causes blood-sugar levels to climb too high. Also, with the body's insulin levels low, fat cells release compounds that are converted to acids called ketones. A buildup of ketones can lead to a condition called ketoacidosis, which is very dangerous and requires emergency treatment.

To remain healthy, people with type 1 diabetes must have insulin injections, usually at least twice a day. This replacement insulin works like the body's own natural insulin to enable normal metabolism and prevent hyperglycemia. It unlocks the cells, permitting glucose to enter them and suppressing the liver's overproduction of glucose. Most critically, it also allows the body to metabolize glucose for energy rather than tapping its reserves of fat.

Though scientists do not yet know for certain what prompts the body's immune system to attack the isulin-producing beta cells, they have identified several culprits. Type 1 diabetes is often an inherited disease, although the pattern of inheritance is not as obvious as for type 2. People with a family history of type 1 diabetes are at increased risk of developing it, because they inherit certain portions of chromosomes, known as haplotypes. These gene fragments then make the individual susceptible to some trigger—most likely a certain virus. If the trigger is encountered, the immune system attacks the insulin-producing cells in the pancreas and destroys them. However, not all people who inherit these haplotypes get type 1 diabetes, and some people without them do get it. As mentioned above, certain environmental factors also apparently trigger the disease, making the exact genetic risk exceedingly difficult to sort out.

One theory is that certain viruses confuse the body's immune system, instructing it to destroy its insulin-producing cells. For example, type 1 diabetes may be a seasonal disease like influenza and pneumonia, with new cases occurring more often in winter than in summer, and more cases occurring in cold climates than in warm ones. Viruses that may cause type 1 diabetes include rubella (the same virus that causes German measles), CoxsackieB (the virus that causes meningitis and several minor intestinal disorders), the mumps virus, and Epstein-Barr virus. Additional support for the virus theory is that virus antibodies—evidence of an infection—have been found in people who have developed type 1 diabetes.

Gestational Diabetes

Pregnant women who have never had diabetes but who have hyperglycemia (high blood-sugar levels) during pregnancy have gestational diabetes. About 4 percent of all pregnant women in the United States—approximately 135,000 women—get gestational diabetes each year.

When a woman has gestational diabetes, her pancreas does not make enough insulin to overcome insulin resistance that occurs during the pregnancy. As with other types of diabetes, this results in hyperglycemia.

The cause of gestational diabetes is not known. The likeliest suspects are hormones released from the placenta—the temporary organ in the mother's body that supports fetal growth. These hormones may block the mother's insulin and cause insulin resistance.

Gestational diabetes usually occurs late in pregnancy, after 24 to 28 weeks. This form of diabetes does not cause the types of birth defects that sometimes occur in babies whose mothers had diabetes before pregnancy. However, gestational diabetes can hurt the fetus by raising its blood-sugar level. Glucose crosses the placenta to the fetus, but insulin does not. The pancreas of the fetus responds by producing more insulin, and then converts the extra glucose to fat.

This can create several problems for the new baby. Because the fetus is getting more glucose than it needs, it stores the excess glucose as fat. A large baby (more than nine pounds) can complicate childbirth and may make the baby susceptible to injury during birth. These babies also have more respiratory problems. In addition, at birth the baby is suddenly deprived of the large supply of sugar provided by the mother, yet the baby may continue to manufacture large amounts of insulin in anticipation of processing it. As a result, the baby may develop low blood-sugar levels shortly after birth, and doctors must then treat the condition. These babies are also at higher risk for obesity and for type 2 diabetes as adults.

Gestational diabetes can be treated to prevent injury to the baby and reduce the need for a caesarean section. Treatment usually involves attention to meal planning and exercise. Sometimes it entails insulin injections for the mother.

Although gestational diabetes usually goes away after pregnancy, once a woman has had this condition the odds are 2 in 3 that she will develop it in future pregnancies. Having gestational diabetes also puts a woman at increased risk of developing type 2 diabetes later in life.

Prediabetes

Prediabetes is a condition in which a person's blood-glucose levels are above normal but are not high enough to qualify as diabetes. Prediabetes is a serious medical condition. It may cause long-term damage to the body, especially the heart and blood vessels, nerve endings, and eyes. However, an important study, the Diabetes Prevention Program, proved that people with prediabetes can prevent or delay type 2 diabetes by practicing good nutrition, controlling their weight, and staying physically active. Exercising 30 minutes a day and losing 5 to 7 percent of body weight, the study showed, reduced the risk of developing type 2 diabetes by 58 percent.

Other Types of Diabetes

Other types of diabetes are quite rare. These include maturity-onset diabetes in the young (MODY), an uncommon form of diabetes that is caused by a single mutation in one or several genes and is usually diagnosed before age 25. Certain ailments can cause diabetes as well. Among them are diseases of the pancreas, some endocrine diseases, and certain genetic diseases, such as Down syndrome or Turner's syndrome. Some medications can cause diabetes, either temporarily or permanently; these include high-dose steroids and drugs used to treat HIV AIDS.

How Many People Have Diabetes?

The number of people with diabetes is increasing rapidly in the United States. In 1990, 4.9 percent of the population had diabetes. By 2001, startlingly, that number had jumped to 7.9 percent. According to the American Diabetes Association and the Centers for Disease Control and Prevention, 20.8 million people in the United States have diabetes: 14.6 million are diagnosed and 6.2 million are undiagnosed. In addition, there are 41 million people with prediabetes. Among Americans age 20 or older, 20.6 million, or 9.6 percent, have diabetes. In the 60 and older age group, 10.3 million, or 20.9 percent, have the disease. In 2005 alone, 1.5 million new cases of diabetes were diagnosed in people aged 20 and older.

Why Is It More Common Today?

Type 2 diabetes is increasing so rapidly in the United States that scientists are calling it an epidemic. Not surprisingly, diabetes is becoming more prevalent in lockstep with another epidemic—that of obesity. Approximately 64 percent of U.S. adults are overweight and 30 percent are obese. Being overweight or obese is the major risk factor for type 2 diabetes.

Although type 2 diabetes has historically been a disease of adults, today children and adolescents are also being diagnosed with it. The

Being overweight or obese puts a person at increased risk for type 2 diabetes and other diseases. Most of us have a sense of whether we weigh too much or not, but sometimes we may think we are overweight when our weight is normal—or vice versa. Scientists have come up with a quick and easy way to tell whether you are underweight, normal weight, overweight, or even obese: a formula called body mass index, or BMI, a calculation of the ratio between your weight and height using a special formula. A BMI below 18.5 indicates you are underweight. A BMI from 18.5 to 24.9 is considered normal, while 25.0 to 29.9 is overweight and 30.0 or above is obese.

To find your BMI, use the chart below or visit the website below, which is maintained by the Centers for Disease Control and Prevention:

www.cdc.gov/nccdphp/dnpa/bmi/calc-bmi.htm

WEIGHT

(lb)	120	130	140	150	160	170	180	190	200	210	220	230	240	250	260	270	280	290	300	310	320
5'0"	23	25	27	29	31	33	35	37	39	41	42	44	47	49	51	53	55	57	59	61	62
5'1"	23	25	26	28	31	33	35	37	39	41	42	44	47	49	51	53	55	57	59	61	62
5'2"	22	24	26	27	29	31	33	35	37	38	40	42	44	46	48	49	51	53	55	57	59
5'3"	21	23	25	27	28	30	32	34	35	37	39	41	43	44	46	48	50	51	53	55	57
5'4"	21	22	24	26	27	29	31	33	34	36	38	39	41	43	45	46	48	50	51	53	55
5'5"	20	22	23	25	27	28	30	32	33	35	37	38	40	42	43	45	47	48	50	52	53
5'6"	19	21	23	24	26	27	29	31	32	34	36	37	39	40	42	44	45	47	48	50	52
5'7"	19	20	22	23	25	27	28	30	31	33	34	36	38	39	40	42	44	45	47	49	50
5'8"	18	20	21	23	24	26	27	29	30	32	33	35	36	38	40	41	43	44	46	47	49
5'9"	18	19	21	22	24	25	27	28	30	31	32	34	35	37	38	40	41	43	44	46	47
5'10"	17	19	20	22	23	24	26	27	29	30	32	33	34	36	37	39	40	42	43	44	46
5'11"	17	18	20	21	22	24	25	26	28	29	31	32	33	35	36	38	39	40	42	43	45
6'0"	16	18	19	20	22	23	24	26	27	28	30	31	33	34	35	37	38	39	41	42	43
6'1"	16	18	19	20	21	22	24	25	26	28	29	30	32	33	34	36	37	38	40	41	42
6'2"	15	17	18	19	21	22	23	24	26	27	28	30	31	32	33	35	36	37	39	40	41
6'3"	15	16	18	19	20	21	23	24	25	26	28	29	30	31	33	34	35	36	38	39	40
6'4"	15	16	17	18	19	21	22	23	24	26	27	28	29	30	32	33	34	35	37	38	39

HEIGHT

My BMI:

Key:
Normal weight   (BMI 19 to 25)
Overweight   (BMI 26 to 29)
Obese   (BMI 30 or over)

_____

increase likely results from the commensurate increase in overweight-ness among youngsters, which in turn stems from high-calorie diets and lack of exercise. This means that complications of diabetes that usually occur only later in life—heart disease, kidney disease, blindness, amputations—may affect these children once they reach their 30s and 40s.

The Urgency of Managing Diabetes

The high blood-sugar levels common to diabetes can damage organs and organ systems in the body. Diabetes puts a person at increased risk for heart disease, stroke, kidney disease, high blood pressure, blindness, nervous-system disease, amputations, dental disease, pregnancy complications, and sexual dysfunction. (The better managed the disease, the less likely these complications.)

There is also a stealth factor: Diabetes can damage the body silently. For this reason, people with diabetes must control their disease carefully through a combination of meal planning, exercise, and, when necessary, medication. A 10-year scientific study of people with diabetes showed that keeping blood-sugar levels close to normal greatly reduces the risk of most complications. If you have diabetes, you can work with your health care team to keep your blood sugar within a healthy range. The payoff is a reduction of the following problems.

Eyes

Diabetes increases your risk for certain eye diseases:

• Diabetic retinopathy occurs when blood vessels inside the eye weaken. This leads to blurry, distorted vision and even blindness.
• Glaucoma is an increase in pressure inside the eye. This can cause loss of peripheral (side) vision.
• Cataracts are a clouding of the lens in the eye. This causes blurry, dull vision.

Nerves

Elevated blood sugar can damage nerves (or cause neuropathy) in the following ways:

• Damage to sensory nerves can cause pain, tingling, numbness, or a burning sensation in the feet and hands.

• Damage to involuntary nerves can lead to diarrhea, constipation, or trouble emptying the bladder. This type of nerve damage also can interfere with sexual function. Men may experience erectile dysfunction, and women may have trouble producing vaginal lubrication.

Feet

High blood sugar increases your risk for these foot problems:

• Poor blood flow (circulation) can prevent sores from healing. This can lead to infection, necessitating the amputation of toes, a foot, or more.

• Damaged nerves can cause numbness so that you cannot feel pain, pressure, heat, or cold in the feet. This, in turn, may keep you from noticing a foot problem until it is too late.

Bladder and Kidneys

High blood sugar can make you susceptible to bladder infections. It can also damage the kidneys, reducing the body's ability to eliminate waste products, and it can cause kidney failure. Here's what to be aware of:

• Urinary-tract infections can occur because bacteria in the bladder feed on high urinary sugar and multiply. You may feel a need to urinate often and have pain when you urinate.

• Kidney damage (nephropathy) causes protein to spill into the urine. It can also cause waste products to build up in the blood. This can foster tiredness, loss of appetite, high blood pressure, swelling in the hands and feet, skin problems, mental confusion, and ultimately kidney failure.

Blood Vessels

High blood sugar can damage blood vessels, impeding blood flow. High blood pressure exacerbates the problem. Here are the most common complications:

• Blood-vessel disease (peripheral vascular disease) can occur when blood flow to the legs or feet is blocked. You may feel weakness, pain, or cramping when you stand or move. The skin may break down and fail to heal.

• Angina or heart attack can occur when blood flow to the heart is blocked. You may feel pressure, tightness, aching, or pain in your chest, jaw, neck, back, or arm. You could even die suddenly.

• Stroke can occur when blood flow to the brain is blocked or when a blood vessel in the brain tears. The is little advance warning; stroke symptoms come on suddenly. Symptoms can include numbness or weakness in the face, arm, or leg; trouble seeing; dizziness or trouble walking; or a sudden, severe headache with no apparent cause. Strokes can cause permanent paralysis, and they can be fatal.

Living Well with Diabetes

Because diabetes is a lifelong disease, managing it is a lifelong responsibility. It does not have to derail your life, however. People with diabetes must take special care of themselves, but they can still travel, play sports, and eat the foods they like.

Working with your health care team—your doctor, your diabetes educator, and your dietitian—you can continue to enjoy a full, active, and healthy life. The chapters that follow explain much more about diabetes, with a special focus on how to cope with the various problems that a person with diabetes is likely to encounter.

2 Diagnosis and Treatment Planning

Discovering you have diabetes can make you feel like you've been hit by a truck. Everything that once seemed easy suddenly becomes complex. You have to think about what you eat. You have to take care of yourself in ways you never considered before. You have to be aware of how well your body is running even if you feel just fine. You have to pay attention to your eyes, skin, and feet far more carefully than in the past. Then there's the business of monitoring your blood-sugar levels and possibly taking insulin or other medications. Where do you begin?

That old saying about taking life one day at a time is good advice at a time like this. Give yourself a break. Take some time to step back and assess your lifestyle. Think what positive impacts you can make on your overall health—your heart, your blood pressure, and your weight. Given the stakes, will eating a balanced, healthy diet be so difficult? Given the benefits, will exercise be such a burden? In addition to being good for your entire body, exercise can be fun: What about taking a walk every day—perhaps with a neighbor or friend you don't get to see very often? You might even think about taking a walk with your spouse or partner—quality time to talk and enjoy each other's company. Eating properly and exercising regularly can help everyone stay healthy. You simply have more of a reason now to take those steps.

The Diagnosis

You've gone for an annual checkup. Or you haven't been feeling so well and went to your health care provider to find out why. Maybe you consulted your doctor for a skin lesion or an injury that wasn't healing properly, and he or she checked your blood-sugar levels. Then came the news that you have diabetes.

Your reaction to that diagnosis may have run a gamut of emotions— fear, anger, denial. At a time like this, it's difficult to consider yourself among the lucky. Still, whatever got you to the doctor's office was a good thing: If you have diabetes that has not yet been diagnosed, high blood-glucose levels may be damaging your body. If your diabetes has been diagnosed, on the other hand, you can control your disease, avoid health problems, make some positive adjustments to your lifestyle, and live a healthy life.

Why You Were at Risk for Diabetes

Health care providers normally screen for diabetes if you are 45 years old or older. If you are also overweight, you need to be especially certain to get tested: Excess weight increases your risk for type 2 diabetes—even at a much younger age.

In addition to older age and being overweight, several other factors can make you more prone to type 2 diabetes:

- You have a parent, brother, or sister with diabetes.
- Your family background is Alaska Native, American Indian, African American, Hispanic American, Asian American, or Pacific Islander.
- You had gestational diabetes or gave birth to at least one baby weighing more than nine pounds.
- You have polycystic ovary syndrome. This health problem affects a woman's menstrual cycle, fertility, hormones, insulin production, heart, and blood vessels.
- Previous blood tests have indicated that you have prediabetes, a condition that is also called either impaired fasting glucose (IFG) or impaired glucose tolerance (IGT).
- You have had other health problems associated with insulin resistance, such as pancreatitis or a condition such as multiple sclerosis or a kidney transplant that requires you to take steroid medications.

If you are younger than 45, are overweight, and have any of the risk factors listed above, consider getting tested for diabetes. Ask your health care provider for a fasting blood-sugar measurement so you will know your status.

How These Risk Factors Work

Knowing what puts you at increased risk for diabetes may suffice for you to modify the risk factors within your control—chiefly being overweight, leading a sedentary lifestyle, and eating a poor diet. Those modifications, in turn, may lower your overall risk. But some people want to know more. They want to understand why a certain condition, such as weight or heredity, makes them more apt to develop the disease. Here is some background to deepen your understanding.

Weight

The single most important risk factor for type 2 diabetes is being overweight. However, not all people with type 2 diabetes are overweight. Some people who think they are overweight actually have a healthy weight, whereas others who are a bit over their healthy weight do not realize it. The best way to figure out whether you are overweight—and, if so, by how much—is to calculate your body mass index (BMI) using the chart on page 12. Don't panic if this table indicates you're a good deal over the desired weight. Studies have shown that you can reduce your risk of type 2 diabetes (as well as your risk of other chronic diseases) by getting closer to your ideal weight. For many people, that requires losing only 5 to 7 percent of your current weight; for others, it requires much more.

Age

As with so many other health problems, the risk for type 2 diabetes increases as you age. Half of all people diagnosed with type 2 diabetes are over 55. You can't do anything about your age, of course, so if you're over 45—the age at which annual screening typically begins—the wisest course of action is to reduce any other risk factors you may have.

Family history

Just as you can't change your age, you can't rewrite your family history. Scientists have discovered a genetic component to diabetes—the disease, especially type 2, runs in families—and some day they may also uncover how to manipulate the genes responsible for the disease. In the meantime, tell your health care provider if any family members have (or had) diabetes.

How much does family history increase your risk? If you have one relative (brother, sister, or parent) with diabetes, your risk of developing type 2 diabetes at some point doubles. If you have two relatives, your risk quadruples.

Race or ethnicity

People with certain ethnic or racial backgrounds are at higher risk of developing type 2 diabetes. These include:

- American Indians
- Hispanic Americans
- African Americans
- Pacific Islanders
- Alaska Natives
- Asian Americans

Compared with non-Hispanic whites, African Americans have twice the risk; Hispanic Americans, 2.5 times the risk; Alaska Natives, 2.5 times the risk; and Native Americans, 5 times the risk. (Precisely how much higher the risk is among Asian Americans has not yet been determined.) If you share any of these ethnicities, you should try to reduce the risk factors that are under your control.

Exercise

Exercise is a key to preventing diabetes. And whether you have diabetes or not, it is also key to maintaining your overall health. Among its many benefits, exercise is good for your heart, your blood pressure, and your weight. For many of us, lack of exercise is an even bigger problem than following a healthy diet. Why?

Many lifestyles in the United States seem to discourage exercise. Whether we're heading to work, school, or the grocery store, the vast majority of us drive just about every place we have to go. Over the past several decades, American neighborhoods and cities have evolved to accommodate the automobile. Indeed, some new suburban neighborhoods lack sidewalks altogether. So how do you get exercise?

It's not complicated. Try walking or some other type of exercise, such as ballroom dancing, tennis, swimming, or jogging. Whatever you choose, pick an exercise you enjoy, then make it part of your routine. Try to exercise five times a week for at least 20 minutes at a time. If it's been a while since you last exercised or if you have health problems, check with your doctor before you start an exercise program.

Exercise is a good way to help prevent diabetes, but it can be useful even if you already have the disease.

First of all, exercise, combined with diet, is an important component of losing weight—an essential goal for most diabetics.

Second, exercise can help you control your blood sugar and the problems caused when it rises too high. Here's a little background on how this mechanism works: Exercise moves sugar into your muscle cells independent of the glucose-ferrying role played by insulin. For that reason, exercise actually lowers your blood sugar even when insulin levels are low. In addition, exercise stimulates two desirable states that are often reduced in people with diabetes: blood flow and vascular patency (the latter is simply the medical term for unclogged blood vessels).

Meal plan

Meal planning is crucial not only for controlling diabetes but also for preventing it. First and foremost, you need to limit your intake of so-called "simple carbohydrates"—that is, sugars that cause a rapid rise in blood glucose. (Complex carbohydrates, because they are digested more slowly, reach the bloodstream more gradually.)

Although carbohydrates and proteins can both be fattening when eaten in excess amounts, the key food ingredient to target for anyone who needs to lose weight is fats. Not only are saturated fats bad for your heart, but being overweight or obese—no matter what foodstuff caused the condition in the first place—is a risk factor for type 2 diabetes.

Studies show that a diet high in saturated fats and trans fats—that is to say, vegetable oils hardened into margarine or shortening—interferes with insulin production. Such a regimen can therefore be a risk factor for type 2 diabetes. Conversely, research has revealed that a diet high in magnesium—found in nuts, whole grains, and leafy green vegetables—can actually reduce your risk of type 2 diabetes.

Gestational diabetes

If you had gestational diabetes while you were pregnant, you are at increased risk of developing type 2 diabetes. About 40 percent of women who had gestational diabetes develop type 2 diabetes within 15 years of that pregnancy.

Even if you didn't have gestational diabetes when you were pregnant, giving birth to a baby that weighed nine pounds or more puts you at increased risk for type 2 diabetes. Large babies are often the result of high blood sugars in the mother. For this reason, you should have an annual fasting blood-sugar check if you had a large baby.

Symptoms

Diabetes can sneak up on you. In its early stages, you may experience no symptoms or you may not recognize them as such. You may feel tired and run down, find yourself having to urinate much more often than usual, or have an excessive thirst. Maybe a cut on your foot is taking a long time to heal, or you've had many more infections than is normal for you.

So how do you know you have diabetes?

Your health care provider can detect the disease early through a medical history and blood tests. Caught early, diabetes can be managed to help prevent complications such as heart, kidney, nerve, blood vessel, or eye disease. Regular screenings for diabetes are therefore crucial, especially if you have any of the risk factors described in this chapter. Listed below are some symptoms that may indicate you have diabetes:

- Frequent urination (polyurea)
- Excessive thirst (polydipsia)
- Unexplained weight loss
- Extreme hunger (polyphagia)
- Blurry vision
- Tingling or numbness in hands or feet
- Excessive fatigue
- Sores that are slow to heal

Keep your risk factors in mind and be alert to any of these symptoms. Regular checkups are always important, but they are especially critical for people with risk factors for diabetes.

Preventing Diabetes

Of the 20.8 million people with diabetes in the United States, 90 to 95 percent have type 2 diabetes. This type is linked to several different risk factors, but you can exert control over two of the most important: body weight and exercise. Although exercise alone cannot ward off diabetes in people of normal weight, it may help them control their blood sugar and manage complications if they have diabetes already. When it is used to promote weight loss, however, exercise can be a critical factor in preventing diabetes.

What Science Says about Preventing Type 2 Diabetes

Can type 2 diabetes be prevented? The answer to this question may help stem the growing epidemic of type 2 diabetes in the United States and other Western countries.

With funding from the U.S. government, scientists studied 3,234 people at high risk for type 2 diabetes in a three-year clinical trial called the Diabetes Prevention Program. All participants in the study were overweight and had high blood-glucose levels (prediabetes). Half of them belonged to higher-risk groups: African American, American Indian, Asian American, Pacific Islander, and Hispanic.

The Diabetes Prevention Program divided participants into groups to study competing approaches for prevention. One group exercised moderately (about 30 minutes a day) and ate a low-fat, low-calorie diet. A second group took a diabetes drug called metformin. A third group took a placebo (a pill with no active ingredients).

The study showed that it is possible to prevent or delay type 2 diabetes. People in the diet-and-exercise group lost 5 to 7 percent of their body weight and cut their risk of getting diabetes by 58 percent. Those in the group taking metformin also cut their risk, but by only 31 percent. Those in the placebo group did not cut their risk at all.

The unassailable conclusion: Diet and exercise are effective in preventing type 2 diabetes. That may sound like a simple nostrum, but empirical evidence—the medical term for bitter experience—shows that only a small percentage of people are able to 1) lose weight and keep it off and 2) start exercising and hew to a workout routine. Also keep in mind that a self-imposed diet/exercise regimen may be more difficult to observe than one you work out with a nutritionist, exercise physiologist, or other health care provider.

Lose a Little, Help a Lot

All of us would like to reach and maintain our ideal weight, but shedding the pounds—especially at 50+—can be a challenge. Although you should aim for a normal weight based on your BMI (see box, page 12), the Diabetes Prevention Program showed that losing even a little weight dramatically reduces your risk of diabetes. For example, if you weigh 200 pounds and are overweight, losing as little as 10 pounds (5 percent of your weight) reduces your risk somewhat. The closer you come to your ideal weight, the more likely you are to avoid becoming diabetic.

Your health care provider can help with advice about exercise. He or she can also refer you to a dietitian or educator who can help you plan flavorful meals. And remember that it isn't only diabetes that exercise and diet help prevent or control. Heart disease, stroke, and several cancers are also related to excessive weight and lack of exercise. So while you're preventing diabetes (or controlling the disease if you already have it), you're also taking positive steps toward overall good health.

A Family Affair

Because diabetes runs in families, preventing the disease can be a family affair. If you're overweight and not eating a healthy diet, chances are that other family members are equally remiss. By working together to get regular exercise and to plan tasty and nutritious meals, you can help your entire family look better, feel better, stay healthy, and prevent health problems.

Testing for Diabetes

As part of your regular physical examination, your health care provider checks your overall health. If you are over age 45 or if you are younger and have risk factors for diabetes, he or she should check you for the disease. Ask your health care provider to administer a diabetes test. Make sure he or she knows about your risk factors, such as a family history of diabetes or the other risk factors listed on page 18.

One routine test for diabetes is the fasting plasma-glucose test—a blood test administered when you have gone at least eight hours without eating, preferably first thing in the morning. This test can detect signs of diabetes or prediabetes.

The doctor will tell you what the results of the test are by giving you a number. Below are the numbers and what they mean.

• 99 and below: Your results are normal. You don't have diabetes or prediabetes.

• 100 to 125: You have a form of prediabetes called impaired fasting glucose (IFG). You are more likely to develop diabetes than people whose blood-glucose levels are 99 or below. Some people with fasting glucose of 100 to 125 may already have diabetes.

• 126 and above: You may have diabetes and will need additional testing.

Sometimes, if your results are normal, your health care provider won't share them unless you ask. So by all means, ask! You want to know where you stand and how you are doing with reducing your risk.

If your fasting plasma-glucose test is above normal, your health care provider will either repeat the test on a different day or order another test called an oral glucose-tolerance test.

Oral Glucose-Tolerance Test

An oral glucose-tolerance test measures your blood glucose in two steps. First you have a blood test in the morning after you have gone at least eight hours without eating. Then you drink a beverage that contains 75 grams of glucose and have another blood test two hours later. The oral glucose-tolerance test isn't as convenient as the fasting plasma-glucose test, but it is more sensitive.

If you have an oral glucose-tolerance test, compare your two-hour values to these:

- 139 and below: Your blood-glucose levels are normal.

- 140 to 199: You have a form of prediabetes called impaired glucose tolerance.

- 200 or above: You may have diabetes. Your health care provider will repeat the test on another day. If your levels are again 200 or above, you have diabetes.

With oral glucose-tolerance tests becoming increasingly rare, some doctors now prefer to measure the blood chemical called hemoglobin A1C. People without diabetes generally have hemoglobin A1C levels below 6. This test should not be used to make a diagnosis, but as a screen for diabetes.

Random Plasma-Glucose Test

Another—and, quite frankly, less reliable—test that checks for diabetes is the random plasma-glucose test. This blood test does not require you to fast beforehand. If the results of the random plasma-glucose test are 200 or above and you have any symptoms of diabetes, you might need to take either a fasting plasma-glucose test or an oral glucose-tolerance test on another day to confirm the diagnosis. If your random plasma-glucose test results are over 120 to 140 but not quite 200, the diagnosis is not clear and other tests will be needed.

Testing for Gestational Diabetes

If you are pregnant, you will have either a fasting plasma-glucose test or a random plasma-glucose test. If either test shows glucose levels above normal, you will need to take a type of oral glucose-tolerance test that is used to diagnose gestational diabetes.

All women should also be tested at 24 to 28 weeks of pregnancy with a glucose test one hour after drinking 50 grams of a glucose drink or three hours after drinking 100 grams of a glucose drink. (A glucose value of 140 mg/dL or greater on the one-hour test requires follow-up with the three-hour test.) This test is similar to the oral glucose-tolerance test described above, except that your blood glucose is checked four times during the test instead of only twice. If your blood-glucose levels are above normal two or more times during the test, you have gestational diabetes.

Your Diabetes Health Care Team

You are the most important member of your diabetes health care team. You are the one who knows best how you feel and how you're doing from day to day. You're the one responsible for what you eat and how much you exercise. You also take the diabetes medications or insulin, and you monitor your own blood-glucose levels. Finally, you're the one who notices when you're not feeling well.

Don't forget that your family and close friends may be part of the team too. They will help and support you in your efforts to lose weight, eat properly, exercise, and monitor your blood sugars.

Then there are your health care providers. Chances are you already have something like a health care team. You see a primary care provider for regular medical examinations and for medical care if you get sick. If you're a woman, you see a gynecologist once a year for an examination. If you're a man, you see a urologist for a prostate exam. And most of us visit an eye doctor (ophthalmologist or optometrist) to have our eyes checked. Perhaps you've never thought of this group of health care providers as a team, but that's what they are.

For people with diabetes, the health care team comprises many of these same members, but it also includes some new ones that you haven't seen before. Why do you need these additional team members?

Because diabetes puts you at risk for several other disorders or complications. Some of these are cardiovascular disease (heart disease, stroke, and circulation problems), eye disease, nerve damage, foot problems, mouth infections, and kidney disease. With the proper care, these health issues can be avoided or prevented. That's why you need specialists to help you evade these complications—or to manage them if they do occur.

Your Primary Care Provider

Think of your primary care provider as your health team leader. He or she will provide your main care but may draft special team members as needed. You may see a family physician, internist, endocrinologist (a doctor with special training in diabetes), or diabetes nurse specialist for your main diabetes care. If you don't see an endocrinologist, try to see a family physician or internist with experience in treating people with diabetes.

If you have diabetes and are working with a health care provider for the first time, you'll want answers to many questions.

First there are the basic queries, such as how comfortable you are with the provider and how much he or she puts you at ease when discussing your lifestyle. You'll want to find out about insurance issues and billing, and you'll want to know how to reach medical help in an emergency. Additionally, who will provide coverage when the doctor is away?

Then there are questions more closely related to your diabetes, such as how much experience and training the provider has had in treating people with diabetes and whether that experience25 is mostly with type 1 or type 2 (or with both). Your primary care provider will be responsible for referring you to specialists for any problems, so you should also find out if he or she is connected with other diabetes specialists who can join your health care team. Also confirm if your primary care provider will refer you to a dietitian (for help with meal planning) and to a nurse or diabetes educator (for help with glucose monitoring and with taking medication or insulin injections, among other issues).

After you've met with your new health care provider, you can decide how you feel about working with him or her. Did the health care provider listen well? Did he or she answer your questions and concerns?

Diabetes Nurse Specialist

If you have just been diagnosed with diabetes (or even if you've had it for some time), you probably have questions about how best to care for yourself. The diabetes nurse specialist (also called a nurse educator) on your health care team is there to answer those questions and to teach you how to take care of yourself.

A nurse educator is either a registered nurse or a nurse practitioner— a registered nurse who has completed advanced coursework and is specially trained to work in diagnosis and treatment. A nurse educator can help you learn how to:

- Use your diabetes medications
- Handle insulin and give yourself insulin shots
- Monitor and record your blood-glucose levels
- Recognize symptoms of high blood glucose (hyperglycemia)
- Recognize symptoms of low blood glucose (hypoglycemia)
- Handle days when you are very sick
- Manage gestational diabetes
- Deal with your emotional concerns
- Avoid skin and other infections

Registered Dietitian

If you have diabetes, your diet is critical in managing your disease. You will probably want to learn how to plan healthy meals and prepare food that is tasty and appealing; nutritious; and low in sugars, other carbohydrates, and fats. Ask if your primary care provider will refer you to a registered dietitian, an important member of your health care team.

A registered dietitian has training in nutrition and has passed a national examination to qualify for that title. You should seek a referral from your doctor to a registered dietitian who specializes in diabetes. He or she will help you assess which foods you should eat or avoid to reach your desired weight, maintain healthy blood-glucose levels, and meet other health goals, such as lowering your cholesterol levels or your blood pressure.

Although there is scant data to support much if any change in nutritional needs as we age, recommended diets for people with diabetes change over time. Even those individuals who have had diabetes for some time can therefore benefit from consulting periodically with a dietitian.

When you contact a dietitian, he or she will help you with more than simple meal planning. The dietitian will explain how certain foods affect your blood-sugar levels and how to read food labels to determine the percentage of certain nutrients a packaged item contains. The dietitian will help you plan meals for a day when you may not feel like eating your usual foods (thus risking low blood glucose, or hypoglycemia). If you exercise vigorously, you will need to learn how to balance your food intake with your level of activity to prevent hypoglycemia. If you use insulin, you will need to learn how to adjust your insulin dosage to what you have eaten and the amount of exercise you are getting. This is especially important for athletes, who burn a lot of calories.

Meal planning can be a challenge, especially at first. Here as well, the dietitian will be a big help. He or she can guide you in learning about portion sizes and types of food to eat, and can recommend recipes or cookbooks. You need not relinquish eating out just because you have diabetes. The dietitian can show you how to order from various restaurant menus and create a plan that will help you reach your goals.

Eye Doctor

Everyone needs an eye doctor to care for vision problems and eye disorders and diseases. But the eye doctor is especially important for someone with diabetes. Having diabetes puts you at risk for certain eye diseases that can cause serious health and vision problems, including blindness (page 13).

Your eye doctor may be an ophthalmologist (a medical doctor who diagnoses and treats eye diseases and performs eye surgery) or an optometrist (a doctor of optometry who tests vision and diagnoses vision problems and eye diseases). For many people with diabetes, it is best to see an ophthalmologist rather than an optometrist. That's because the changes that often take place in the retina (the back of the eye) in people with diabetes may require treatment that only an ophthalmologist can perform.

Whichever type of doctor you select, you should see your eye doctor for an examination at the time of diagnosis of type 2 diabetes and at least once a year. If you have an eye disorder that needs to be checked more frequently, of course, your eye doctor will increase the frequency of your appointments. Your eye doctor will refer you to a specialist if you develop any of the eye complications of diabetes.

Podiatrist

Simply put, a podiatrist is a foot specialist with special training in caring for the feet and lower legs. People with diabetes often need a podiatrist because they are at risk for foot problems arising from possible nerve damage, circulation problems, and increased risk of infection. Combined, all three conditions can bring on foot problems—especially infections—that quickly become severe.

You should report any foot problem—a sore, cut, infection, or other injury—to your primary care physician or podiatrist immediately. By seeking treatment for such an issue right away, you may ward off a severe infection that could lead to gangrene and the loss of toes—or even a foot or lower leg.

In addition to treating foot problems such as ingrown toenails, calluses, or corns, your podiatrist is responsible for foot maintenance. Many doctors warn people with diabetes not to trim their own toenails; the danger of injury or infection when doing so is too high to tolerate. The podiatrist can do this for you.

Dentist

Everyone needs to see a dentist for checkups and tooth care. Because diabetes can cause certain mouth problems, people with the condition may require extra dental care.

Excess blood sugar in the mouth makes it easier for bacteria to thrive. This can open the door to gum and other mouth infections. The excess sugar can also make you more prone to cavities. To prevent these problems, see your dentist every six months. Be sure to tell him or her you have diabetes so that the dentist can be especially attentive to problem signs. And ask about using a fluoride mouthwash or toothpaste.

Exercise Specialist

Exercise not only helps prevent diabetes, it can help you manage the disease if you do have it. Exercise can lower your blood-sugar levels and help your body use insulin more efficiently. It also helps with weight control, cholesterol levels, blood pressure, and stress. It can help improve the circulation to your legs and strengthen your heart.

A specialist known as an exercise physiologist can help you develop an exercise plan that works for you. An exercise physiologist is a health care professional with training in the science of exercise who has degrees or graduate training in exercise physiology. Many exercise physiologists are certified by the American College of Sports Medicine. Not everyone with diabetes needs an exercise specialist, however, so ask your doctor before pursuing this route.

Don't Neglect Your Emotional Health

If you have just been diagnosed with diabetes, or even if you've had it for a while, the stress of managing your disease can be overwhelming. Besides taking a personal toll, it can affect your relationships with family members and others. Tending to the needs of your body is therefore not enough. You also must care for your mind and your emotional health. A mental-health professional can help you cope.

Many types of mental-health professionals can provide counseling. To find the right one for you, ask your primary care provider to make a referral based on your particular need:

• Social worker: A mental-health professional, ideally with a Master in Social Work (MSW) degree, who provides individual, group, or family therapy.

• Clinical psychologist: A psychologist trained in individual, group, and family counseling.

• Psychiatrist: A medical doctor who provides counseling and can also prescribe medicine to treat emotional problems.

• Marriage and family therapists: Social workers, psychologists, or psychiatrists with special training in marriage and family problems. They can help relieve the stresses that diabetes invariably exerts on families and personal relationships.

3 Managing Diabetes

Y ou've been diagnosed with diabetes. Your health care providers have told you about the lifestyle changes you will want to make to live with diabetes and remain healthy. You have a fistful of brochures, instructions from your health care team about diet and exercise, perhaps some prescriptions for diabetes medication, and possibly insulin. If you're like many people, you're probably on information overload at this point. Or you may be having trouble deciding what to do next: How exactly does one live day to day with diabetes?

Because you are the one in charge of your ongoing care, this chapter aims to provide a thorough understanding of the choices you face in taking care of yourself. This information is intended to bolster, not replace, the advice and support of your health care team—the group of health care professionals available to provide advice and answer your questions.

Because you have diabetes, as you probably know by now, your body's system for automatically producing and managing the hormone insulin is not working properly. This means that insulin is not keeping the glucose levels in your blood in a healthy range. Controlling blood glucose is vital to your health and well-being.

What happens now?

Whether you have type 2 or type 1 diabetes, managing this disease means maintaining your blood-glucose levels as near normal as possible. How you do that differs depending on what type of diabetes you have. For people with type 2 diabetes, your treatment will involve exercise and weight control, as well as possibly oral medication or insulin injections. If you have type 1, insulin replacement through injections, meal planning, and exercise is the basis for managing diabetes.

Such and more are the ground rules for managing diabetes. You will want to closely monitor what's going on in your body and how you feel. You'll need to recognize the signs that mean your glucose levels are out of kilter so that you can adjust food intake or medication doses. If you're exercising heavily, for example, your blood-glucose levels may fall lower than they should. Or if you're sick or stressed, your blood-sugar levels may rise.

Here's the kernel of what you need to remember: Managing diabetes is a balancing act. You'll have to train yourself to monitor the functions that your body once handled on its own. At first you'll have to work hard at this, but eventually it will become easier. (Don't expect the habit ever to become completely axiomatic, though; as Thomas Jefferson said of freedom, it requires eternal vigilance.) By working with your health care team, you will learn to read the signals that your body sends you.

Managing Means Planning

Managing your diabetes effectively takes planning. What you eat and when, how often and how vigorously you exercise all relate to what is going on with your body's blood-glucose levels. If you are overweight, you will need to work with your health care team to develop a plan for reducing your weight. If you are at a healthy weight, you will want to keep it that way. So meal planning and exercise are key to diabetes management. You will also need to check or "monitor" your blood-glucose levels regularly. Finally, if your meal plan and exercise don't keep your blood-sugar levels normal or near normal, your health care provider may prescribe a medication, or even insulin injections, to help bring those levels under control. If you have type 1 diabetes, insulin will be a mainstay of your diabetes-management plan.

Meal Planning

Diet is a crucial part of managing diabetes. Not only is it important to eat the right foods, but you need to develop a regular schedule for eating. When you eat at the same times each day, you set a pattern for your body. When you deviate from your regular schedule, by contrast, you may need to adjust your medications. If you take insulin, eating regularly will make it easier to balance the amount of insulin you take against the amount of food your body turns into energy. You can then collaborate with your health care provider to rough out a schedule for taking insulin before eating. This in turn should help you keep your blood-glucose levels in a healthy equilibrium.

A meal plan will ease the task of scheduling meals. A plan gives you guidelines for the types and amounts of food you should eat—and when to eat them. Working with your dietitian, you can develop a flexible plan that works for you and includes many foods that you like.

Exercise

Being active helps you control your weight, lower your blood pressure, and lower your cholesterol levels—three sure ways to minimize the risk of cardiovascular disease, among other ailments. Exercise also strengthens your muscles and bones. To top it all off, it's a great way to defuse stress. Losing weight and getting regular exercise can help most people with type 2 diabetes bring their blood glucose to normal levels—sometimes to levels that don't require medication.

When you exercise, your body demands energy. First it draws on your circulating glucose—that is, the glucose available in your bloodstream. If the right amount of insulin is available in your blood, the system works normally and the insulin ferries glucose into your muscle cells. If the right amount of insulin is not available, on the other hand, only a little glucose makes its way into your muscle cells, forcing those cells to seek out other sources of the precious, energy-rich commodity. First they draw on glycogen—the form in which carbohydrate is stored in muscle cells. Glycogen reserves don't last very long, however, so when insulin is scarce the muscles soon run out of energy. Faced with this potentially catastrophic deficit, the body is forced to metabolize (or burn) fat as an emergency source of energy—a good thing in small doses, but a poisonous proposition in large doses. (For more about "killer fat," see "Diabetic Ketoacidosis" on pages 41–42.)

Although exercise is good, it can lower your blood-glucose levels to the point of **hypoglycemia,** especially if you take insulin or certain diabetes medications. (*Hypoglycemia* is a condition in which your blood-sugar levels fall very low. For a full list of its symptoms, see the box on page 43; chapter 10 also gives a detailed explanation of hypoglycemia—and the importance of treating it promptly.) If you exercise just after an insulin injection, your muscles may take in more glucose than usual. Or your body may absorb the insulin more quickly, especially if it was injected near a muscle you're using intensively in the exercise. For these reasons, it's critical to monitor your blood-sugar levels and adjust your diet and insulin as needed. Work with your health care providers to learn how to achieve this.

The best time to exercise is when your blood-glucose levels are at their highest—usually one to three hours after eating. Test your blood sugar before you begin to exercise. If it's below 120 mg/dL, eat a snack containing some carbohydrate (this will be listed on the package) or eat some fruit; the idea behind this remedy is to raise your blood glucose enough to avoid hypoglycemia (see box, page 43.) Test the level again 30 minutes later to make sure it's not too low. Carry some food or glucose tablets with you just in case you begin to feel symptoms of hypoglycemia. If you are doing a particularly heavy workout, be certain to check your blood glucose once you finish exercising. Chapter 8 discusses exercise and its effect on blood-glucose levels in more detail.

Monitoring Your Blood-Glucose Levels

If you have diabetes, you need to monitor your blood-glucose levels to know how these levels change throughout the day—especially in response to exercise or to certain foods. You need to determine if you're taking too much (or not enough) oral medication or insulin. People with type 2 diabetes generally need not check their blood-glucose levels as often as those with type 1. Checking your blood frequently helps you tailor your treatment—oral medication, insulin, meal planning, and exercise—to fit your individual needs. Work with your health care providers to determine how often you should check your glucose levels, and to establish target blood-glucose levels.

Blood-glucose levels vary throughout the day. If your blood sugar dips too low or spikes too high, you may not notice it right away. Regular monitoring gives you a continuous read on your blood-glucose level and helps you keep it near normal. It also helps you adjust your insulin doses, and it will keep your doctor apprised of whether your oral medications are at the right dosage and frequency. Monitoring and adjusting can also help prevent hypoglycemia.

Various devices are available for monitoring blood glucose. Chapter 4 discusses the options in greater detail and explains how to use each one.

Medications for Type 2 Diabetes Help Control Blood-Glucose Levels

Often meal planning and exercise fail to control blood-glucose levels for people with type 2 diabetes. If this happens, your health care provider may prescribe an oral medication—a pill—to help keep these levels near normal. These medications are available in a number of different "classes," and they have different actions to help you control your diabetes. Some drugs stimulate your pancreas to make more insulin, for instance. Others signal the liver to decrease its production of glucose. One class of drugs lowers the absorption of the carbohydrates you eat, while others help insulin work more efficiently. A drug in any class can be taken alone or in combination with other diabetes medications. Oral medications for type 2 diabetes are discussed at greater length in Chapter 6.

If oral medications don't work for you—or if you have a bad reaction to one of them—your doctor may prescribe insulin injections to help bring your blood sugar back under control. Some people use both oral medication and insulin.

Insulin

Several types of insulin are available for "replacement treatment," as it is called; your health care provider will help you find the right type or combination for you. Some people with type 2 diabetes use replacement treatment along with diet, exercise, and (occasionally) other diabetes medications. If you have type 1 diabetes, your pancreas is making little or no insulin, so replacement insulin is pivotal to regulating blood-glucose levels. To stay healthy, you must replace the insulin that your body is no longer making.

Replacing insulin means giving yourself insulin injections. Why not an insulin pill? Scientists and medical researchers have yet to invent an insulin dose that can be taken by mouth, because the human digestive system destroys the hormone. Chapter 5 discusses a new form of inhalable insulin that may work for some people with diabetes.

Because insulin needs vary from one person to the next, no single plan works for everyone. Most people with type 1 diabetes must take insulin at least three times a day to keep their blood-glucose levels as close to normal as possible. How often to take insulin—and how much and what type of it to take—will hinge on your own individual needs.

The methods for injecting insulin are multiform: They include syringes (which are used once and discarded), pen injectors (which hold multiple doses), and insulin pumps (which deliver insulin continuously, with additional insulin given as needed at the push of a button). Working with your health care team, you can determine which method works best for you. (Chapter 5 also explores the various types and combinations of insulin—and how they affect your body.)

Other Medications

Just as certain foods can affect your blood-glucose levels, so too can certain medications besides insulin. Inform your health care providers and pharmacist what other medicines you take! These include prescription medications for other health problems; any over-the-counter medications, such as aspirin or cold medicine; any patches or medicated gum, such as smoking-cessation aids; and any vitamins or supplements. This does not mean you must stop taking these medicines; it simply means you should know if, and how, they will affect your blood-glucose levels.

Diabetes Emergencies

The thought of a diabetes emergency is frightening until you learn that most such crises can be easily prevented or resolved.

A diabetes emergency means you have lost control of your blood-glucose levels. If those levels rise too high or fall too low, urgent problems can develop. However, a few simple steps on your part will usually suffice to correct these imbalances. Described below are the symptoms of both high and low blood-glucose levels; you will also find advice on how to prevent an emergency.

Diabetic Ketoacidosis

Extremely high blood-glucose levels (hyperglycemia) can lead to diabetic ketoacidosis, or DKA, the precise mechanism of which is described below. Left untreated, DKA can result in a coma.

DKA is brought on by insulin deficiency. When the body cannot access enough insulin to move glucose into cells (where it is metabolized, or burned, for energy), it instead burns fat as fuel. Fat metabolism produces organic compounds known as ketones, which can accumulate in the blood and make it acidic. This state of affairs is called diabetic ketoacidosis.

DKA occurs when insulin falls to an extremely low level. This drop-off may happen for a number of reasons: Perhaps you missed an injection, or your last dose of insulin was too small. You may have been ill or under unusual stress—both of which spur the body to produce hormones that interfere with the action of insulin. No matter what the precise cause, your blood-glucose levels become very high and ketones build up in your blood.

As ketone and glucose levels rise in your blood, your kidneys swing into action, producing large amounts of urine to flush out those toxic compounds. This triggers dehydration. You may also experience nausea and vomiting—which, in turn, accelerate the dehydration. In the context of advancing DKA, dehydration can represent something far more noxious than merely low body fluids; it can also drive your blood pressure down. Although some people have blood pressure that is always a bit lower than normal, sudden drops in blood pressure can cause heart problems, kidney failure, and shock.

If you have diabetes, especially type 1, be alert to the signs of DKA. One such symptom is fruity breath, generated by the body's effort to offload the ketone acetone through your lungs. Other symptoms include frequent urination, thirst, rapid breathing, nausea, vomiting, fatigue, and abdominal pain. As ketoacidosis advances, the changes in body chemistry can cause confusion and even coma.

DKA does not happen instantly. It progresses over several hours or days, meaning regular glucose monitoring can tell you if you're at risk for it. People with type 2 diabetes rarely have ketoacidosis because their insulin levels rarely fall low enough to trigger the liver to produce ketones. If you have type 1 diabetes and your blood glucose is above 300 mg/dL, you are indeed at risk—and you need to take immediate action to lower your blood sugar. DKA can be treated, usually with extra insulin and intravenous fluids to combat dehydration.

Ask your health care provider if and when you should test for ketones. Testing is done with ketone sticks, which are dipped in a sample of your urine to determine your ketone level. Perform this test whenever your blood-sugar levels become unusually high or if you develop a new illness—particularly one that entails nausea, vomiting, or abdominal pain. If the ketone test shows more than a trace of ketones, take the following action:

- Call your health care provider right away.
- Drink plenty of fluids such as water and clear soups.
- Take steps, as taught and instructed, to lower your blood sugar.

Hypoglycemia

Just as too much glucose in your blood can cause problems, so can too little. This deficit creates a condition known as hypoglycemia (see box, opposite). Your blood sugar may fall because you missed a meal or a snack, because you exercised more than usual, or because you took too much diabetes medication or insulin.

You need to be able to recognize the symptoms of hypoglycemia: If your blood sugar falls too low, your brain won't get enough glucose. You could then pass out and be unable to help yourself. Hypoglycemia can develop very quickly; often it becomes severe within minutes.

You will most likely learn to recognize the symptoms of hypoglycemia immediately and be able to deal with them at once. For added protection, though, tell your friends and co-workers exactly what they should do in the event you become confused or lose consciousness.

When someone with diabetes loses consciousness from hypoglycemia, the quickest way to revive the person is with an injection of

The National Institute of Diabetes and Digestive and Kidney Diseases lists the following main symptoms of hypoglycemia:

- Nervousness and shakiness

- Perspiration

- Dizziness or light-headedness

- Sleepiness

- Confusion

- Difficulty speaking

- Hunger

- Feeling anxious or weak

If you have any of these symptoms, check your blood-sugar level. If it is low (less than about 70, although some people start to experience these sensations around 80), follow this course of action right away:

- Take 15 grams of some fast-acting sugar. This can be three or four glucose tablets; 1 tablespoon of table sugar in water; 4 ounces of fruit juice; or 4 ounces of regular (not diet) soda.

- After 15 minutes, check your blood sugar again. If it is still outside your target range or getting closer, repeat the step above.

- Repeat these steps until your blood-glucose level reaches at least 70. If, after hitting this level, your next meal is an hour or more away, have a snack.

glucagon. People with type 1 diabetes should therefore keep an up-to-date glucagon-injection kit with them at home and at work. The glucagon needs to be mixed immediately before it is used, so explain to family members or co-workers how to mix and administer the injection. If you believe that someone has lost consciousness because of hypoglycemia and you do not have access to glucagon, call 911 and ask for paramedics with intravenous glucose. Never try to force an unconscious person to swallow liquids or solids.

Hyperglycemic Hyperosmolar Nonketotic Syndrome (HHNS)

Hyperglycemic hyperosmolar nonketotic syndrome (HHNS) is a rare emergency condition that occurs when blood glucose rises to extremely high levels—over 600 mg/dL. Unlike diabetic ketoacidosis, there are no ketones present in HHNS. Although anyone with diabetes is susceptible, HHNS is most common in type 2 diabetes and in those over age 60. The condition can result from an illness or an infection, stress, or starting a new medication. When blood-glucose levels get very high, the body starts to rid its excess sugar through urination. Frequent urination leads to dehydration, and as dehydration progresses, the urine turns a dark color. Dehydration can lead to seizures, coma, and death.

HHNS does not occur quickly. It usually develops over the course of several days or even weeks. If you are monitoring your blood sugar regularly, you will be aware if your levels are rising. If the levels rise to 350 mg/dL or higher, call your health care provider. If they are over 500 mg/dL, you should get emergency care immediately, either from your health care provider or by going to an emergency room. HHNS is a very serious condition.

Anyone with diabetes should be alert to the symptoms of HHNS, but if you have type 2—or an elderly relative or friend with the disease—you should be especially alert to its signs:

- Extreme thirst; dry mouth
- Blurred vision
- Hallucinations
- Feeling sleepy or confused
- Weakness on one side of the body
- High fever and/or warm, dry skin

The Big Picture— Managing Your Overall Health

Your health care team is there to help you learn to manage your diabetes and to monitor how well you're doing, not only with blood-sugar control but with your health in general. Your doctor or diabetes nurse will recommend regular checkups, which will include a blood-pressure check and a cholesterol test. These exams will often include an A1C test—a critical blood test that shows your average blood-sugar level for the past two to three months. This enables you and your health care provider to assess how well your treatment plan is working.

Blood Sugar and the A1C

Checking your blood sugar throughout the day provides an important—but limited—measure of how well you are managing your diabetes. Your daily checks are like snapshots of blood-sugar control at any given time. The A1C test, by contrast, reveals a much bigger picture. It measures your average blood-sugar levels over a two- to three-month period, providing a more accurate measure of overall diabetes control.

Your health care provider may suggest having the A1C test twice a year. If your treatment plan changes, you may be tested more often. This simple blood test can be done in your doctor's office, and you needn't fast before taking the test.

Talk with your doctor about your personal A1C goal. You can then work together to find ways of meeting this goal. By lowering your A1C value just 1 percentage point, you greatly reduce the risk for eye, kidney, and nerve problems. In general, if your A1C value is:

• Less than 7 percent, your diabetes treatment plan is working. This helps reduce the risk of health problems. Be sure to get your A1C checked at least twice a year; adjustments in your treatment plan may be needed over time.

• Greater than 7 percent, reducing your blood-sugar levels is a priority. Each point over 7 greatly increases a person's risk for developing diabetes-related complications.

Blood Pressure

Everyone should have her or his blood pressure checked during a checkup, but if you have high blood pressure and type 2 diabetes, you need to control your blood pressure carefully. Be sure to have it checked each time you visit your health care provider. Your goal should be a reading of no more than 130/80. If your blood pressure is higher, your doctor may prescribe medications to lower it.

Cholesterol

Your cholesterol numbers signify your risk for heart disease. A cholesterol test will tell you what your HDL, LDL, and triglyceride levels are. Everyone should get their cholesterol checked regularly, but people with diabetes, who are at increased risk of heart disease, should have theirs checked at least once a year. These are the recommended levels:

- HDL cholesterol—above 40 for men, above 50 for women
- LDL cholesterol—below 100
- Total cholesterol—below 200
- Triglycerides—below 150

Other Tests Your Doctor May Recommend

In addition to gauging cholesterol and blood pressure, your health care provider will check your feet for injuries or signs of nerve damage and perform several other tests to assess your health. These are some other tests that your provider may recommend:

- Serum creatinine—a blood test that evaluates kidney function
- Thyroid hormones—a blood test that evaluates thyroid function
- Electrocardiogram (ECG)—a simple test that records the electrical activity of the heart
- Microalbumin—a urine test for abnormal quantities of protein

The Importance of Immunizations

If you have diabetes, you are more susceptible to many other illnesses—and these ailments may strike you harder. For this reason, it's key that you stay up to date on all your immunizations, especially influenza and pneumonia. Be sure to get annual influenza and pneumonia vaccinations to stave off these diseases (think about getting them in October or early November, before the debut of flu and pneumonia season).

Ask your health care provider what other vaccinations you may need, such as tetanus, diphtheria, or hepatitis. Good prevention is the best protection!

4 Monitoring Your Blood Sugar

Y ou now know that controlling your blood-glucose levels will help you avoid many of the problems associated with diabetes—both long-term complications (see chapter 11) and the more immediate difficulties of hypoglycemia (low blood sugar) and hyperglycemia (high blood sugar). And you are probably becoming more attuned to your body's own signals indicating when your blood-sugar level is either too high or too low.

Still, you need a more precise measurement of your blood sugar for two key reasons: to assess how well your treatment plan is working, and to become even more adept at gauging how you feel versus what your levels are. Even those who are highly attuned to how they feel can benefit from close monitoring, which will help you tighten your control of your blood sugar. Monitoring can also show you how specific food choices and types of exercise affect your blood sugar.

If you use insulin, regular monitoring is particularly important: It allows you to adjust the amount of insulin you are taking. Your health care team will tell you how often you should monitor and how to adjust your insulin doses accordingly.

How Is It Done?

You test or "monitor" your blood-glucose levels with a special device called a glucose meter. Testing is a simple two-step process. First you take a sample of your blood; second, you dab it onto a test strip. Most glucose meters require that the strip be placed in the machine before you dab the blood on it. (If not, you dab the blood, then insert the test strip.) The meter reveals what your blood-sugar level is.

Most glucose meters include a pen-shaped device that holds a spring-loaded lancet—a small, sharp needle. The test proceeds as follows: You put a fresh lancet in the pen, then put a fresh strip in the meter and wait until the meter tells you it has read the strip. (Each meter is calibrated differently, so almost all of them require recalibration with each new package of strips.) You then hold the pen against your finger or forearm, push a button, and the lancet pricks your skin, drawing a small amount of blood. This pricking procedure is virtually painless; even small children become accustomed to the minor sting. Most people find that pricking the forearm is less painful than the fingertip.

After pricking your skin with the lancet, you squeeze a drop of blood onto the special test strip that has been freshly inserted in the meter. You wait five to 30 seconds (each meter is different), whereupon the meter gives you a digital readout of your blood sugar. After removing the strip and throwing it away, you remove the used lancet and discard it as well.

How Often Should You Check Your Glucose?

Your health care team will tell you how often to check your blood glucose. You can check it more often if you like, but be sure to check it at least as many times a day as your health care team recommends. For example, people with type 2 diabetes who are taking pills may be advised by their health care provider to check their blood glucose before different meals or on different days, three or four times a week. Most other people with type 2 diabetes should test their blood glucose before each meal and at bedtime for one week every four to six weeks. Those with type 1 diabetes, those using insulin pumps or on intensive insulin therapy, and women with gestational diabetes should check their blood glucose before and after every meal, and occasionally at 3:00 a.m.

How to Monitor Your Blood Glucose

If you are monitoring your own blood glucose, be sure to read the instructions for the specific type of monitoring kit you're using and follow the directions of your health care team. The list below offers guidance if you're helping someone else, such as a child or elderly family member, or if you just need a general reminder of the steps involved.

1. Get ready

- Wash your hands thoroughly with soap and water; then dry them well.
- Follow the directions for placing a test strip in the meter.

2. Draw a drop of blood

- Put a fresh lancet in the pen, then prick the side of your finger near the tip with the lancet. Squeeze gently until you get a drop of blood.

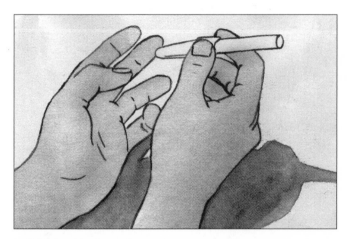

> Prick the side of your finger.

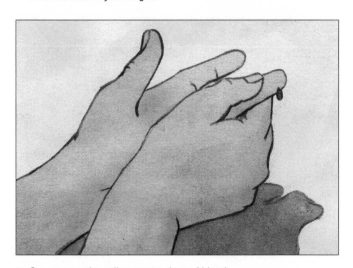

> Squeeze gently until you get a drop of blood.

• Some devices allow blood to be drawn from "alternative sites" such as the heel of the palm, the forearm, or even the thigh. If your device allows you to take blood from another part of your body, follow the directions for doing so. Be sure to wash the skin where you will draw the sample.

•Dispose of the lancet in a special sharps disposal container. (Ask your health care team where you can obtain one.)

3. Place the drop on a strip

• Be sure the meter displays the appropriate message or symbol that it is time to place blood on the strip.

• Apply the drop of blood to the strip according to the directions.

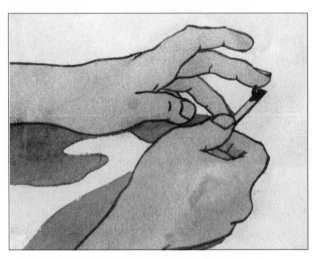

> Place the drop of blood on a strip.

4. Read and record your results

• Wait the specified time for your glucose meter to display the result.

• If you see an error message, start over with a fresh strip and a fresh drop of blood.

• Record the date, time, and reading in the logbook your health care team gave you or in any small notebook. (Take this record to each medical appointment.) Remove the strip and throw it away, then remove the used lancet and throw it away too.

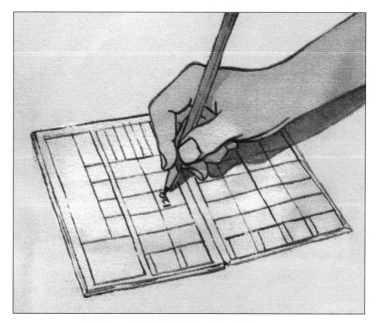

> Record the date, time, and reading in your logbook.

Selecting a Glucose Meter

According to the Food and Drug Administration, more than 25 different brands of blood-glucose meters are now on the market. For people with impaired vision, there are meters with large displays and ones that "talk" so you can hear what your reading is. Most meters record and store a number of test results; some can even be connected to your personal computer, allowing you to transfer your results to a spreadsheet program. Some machines have the lancet built in, enabling you to take your blood sample and test it with the same device.

Most people should have more than one glucose meter on hand, although it is usually best that they all be the same brand. One meter should always be held in reserve as a back-up, though in practice many people have discovered that they prefer to keep one near the bed, a second somewhere else in the house, a third in the office, and a fourth in their purse or briefcase.

Among the crucial factors in deciding which model to buy is size, which varies considerably from one device to the next. One particularly popular glucose meter is disposable: It takes the form of a canister of 50 strips with its own built-in meter, and when the 50 strips are used you simply throw the thing away. No calibration is needed for this model.

Another salient selling point is the speed with which a meter delivers results. Some take as little as five seconds, others as long as 30. Some require more blood on the test strip than others. Most tend to be small enough to carry in a handbag, a briefcase, or even a pocket, and many people have more than one for convenience.

Glucose meters usually cost less than $100. Most insurance plans, including Medicare, cover at least part of the cost of the device, test strips, lancets, the lancing device, batteries for the meter, and cleaning solutions for the meter (though the latter may not be necessary). Check with your insurer to see if the meter you want is covered and how much the company will pay.

Be sure to coordinate your choice with your health care team, which can point you to the best model for your needs. Take your new meter to your next appointment, especially if you need some help learning how to use it. Your health care provider will also compare your meter's results with office tests to ensure accurate readings.

Keep these things in mind when you go shopping for a glucose meter:

• How much blood does the meter need for each test?
• How quickly does the meter deliver results?
• What is the overall size of the meter? Will it fit in a pocket or handbag?
• Can the meter store test results in its memory or connect to your computer?
• How much does the meter cost? Will your insurance company cover all or only part of the cost?
• How much do test strips cost for a given meter? Are generic strips available for that meter? (Test strips are usually the most expensive part of glucose monitoring, and generic strips are less expensive. See "Using generic test strips," page 55.)
• Is the display easy to read?

• Is the packaging of the strips easy for you to open and handle? (Some strips come in canisters, others in foil envelopes. Some are quite difficult for visually impaired people and those with arthritis to open.)

Continuous Glucose Monitoring

Recent developments in glucose monitoring offer people with diabetes another option for managing blood-glucose levels—"bloodless meters," which employ a sensor placed under the skin.

One sensor, the Guardian® RT continuous glucose-monitoring system, displays real-time glucose values every five minutes and alerts patients when glucose levels become too high or too low. A disposable sensor is inserted beneath the skin and transmits your glucose readings via radio frequencies to a display monitor. You can set the threshold to sound an alarm if your glucose levels become potentially dangerous. You can also download readings into a computer and work with your doctor to use these for managing your diabetes. You calibrate the monitor every 12 hours by taking a finger-stick reading with a standard glucose monitor and entering it into the Guardian® RT's monitor. (The same company makes the MiniMed Paradigm, a pump with a continuous sensor. Because the sensor feeds information to the pump, this system has revolutionized the care of type 1 diabetes.)

Another sensor type of continuous glucose monitor, the CGMS System Gold, is designed to help your doctor or health care team manage your diabetes. It is similar to the Guardian® RT in that a sensor inserted under the skin relays glucose readings to a monitor every five minutes. After three days, you and your doctor review the readings the monitor has collected. This helps you both identify hidden patterns in your glucose levels, such as episodes of hypoglycemia, enabling the doctor to adjust your medication or insulin.

A third sensor-type monitoring system is the DexCom™ STS® Continuous Glucose Monitoring System. Like other continuous monitoring systems, it involves inserting a small sensor under the skin. (You can do this yourself, or have your health care provider insert it.)

A wireless transmitter that fits comfortably under your clothing sends glucose readings from the sensor to a small receiver, which can be worn on a belt or carried in a handbag. The sensor is disposable and can be worn for up to three days before being replaced. The DexCom sensor provides continuous monitoring, high- and low-glucose alerts, and trend readings at one-, three-, and nine-hour intervals.

Continuous glucose monitoring systems are designed to be used as supplements to, not replacements for, conventional glucose monitors that require a blood sample. Ask your doctor if you can benefit from the continuous monitoring provided by these devices.

What If a Reading Is Very High or Low?

Given the crucial role of blood-sugar monitoring, it's easy to see why health care professionals place such a premium on guaranteeing accurate glucose readings when those measurements are taken by people with diabetes. Some particularly high or low readings may result from improper use of a meter. Other readings are truly very high or low; these may result from the use of a new meter, or they may show up on the meter of someone who has never gauged his or her blood-sugar levels before—and is stunned to see how elevated or depressed those readings are, in light of the relative absence of symptoms.

The bottom line of all this is: Be sure you know how to use your meter. If you are confident you are using it correctly but doubt the accuracy of a reading, talk to your health care provider about what steps to take next. In the vast majority of cases, you will need only to take a second measurement, using either the same meter or—preferably—another one.

Never forget, of course, that unusually high or low readings may signal hyperglycemia or hypoglycemia. If your first set of unusual results is confirmed by a second, trust it—and take action. Some steps to take are spelled out in Appendix D, "Diabetes Emergencies," which provides guidance on treating hyperglycemia and hypoglycemia.

As you become more aware of your body's own signals, you will learn to know when you have merely a meter problem and when the problem in fact stems from your blood-glucose levels.

Getting It Right

Check your meter often

Because it is so important to know your blood-glucose levels with precision, check your meter regularly to make sure it is working properly; the user's manual will tell you how to do this. You will probably have to adjust or recalibrate your meter periodically. Some kits include—or you can buy separately—a testing solution of a known glucose level that you can use to gauge the accuracy of your meter's readings. Other meters feature a cartridge with a special test strip that checks the meter and emits an electronic signal to let you know it is reading correctly.

Almost all glucose monitors require that you recalibrate the machine whenever you start using a new batch of test strips. (Even strips of the same brand can vary from batch to batch.) The only glucose meter that does not necessitate this reset is the disposable version, which is precalibrated.

Cleaning your meter

Your particular model of meter may or may not need to be cleaned every so often. If it does, you usually do this with soap and water and a soft cloth. Don't use alcohol or cleansers containing alcohol unless the instructions tell you to. Some meters give you an electronic alert when they need cleaning. In some cases, you must return the meter to the manufacturer for a professional cleaning.

Using generic test strips

Generic or third-party test strips are available for many glucose meters. They typically cost less and tend to be just as reliable as the brand recommended by the meter manufacturer. Check the package to be sure the generic strips are designed to be used with your meter. Especially if you have the "new and improved" model of a meter, generics that worked with the old version may no longer be compatible. If for any reason you are uncertain whether generic test strips will work with your meter, call the manufacturer's toll-free number and ask.

New Types of Meters and Lancets

Manufacturers are constantly coming up with new types of blood-glucose meters that obtain results in different ways. You can use any blood-letting device with any brand of meter, but some people are particularly sensitive to finger pricks; makers have therefore developed versions that allow you to take blood samples from different parts of the body.

Invariably, manufacturers will continue to investigate all sorts of alternatives to traditional blood-glucose meters. Seek the advice of your health care team if you'd like to explore other options.

5 When You Need Insulin Therapy

The hormone insulin is an amazing player in the body's complex regulation of its energy supplies. Produced by a collection of cells in the pancreas called beta cells, insulin travels through the bloodstream and acts to move glucose from the blood into the body's cells. There it facilitates the glucose's conversion to energy. It is often said that insulin "makes glucose available" for cells. Indeed, it would not be too much of a stretch to say that insulin is indispensable.

If you have type 2 diabetes, insulin may not be able to do its job properly, or your body may simply not be producing enough. If you have type 1 diabetes, almost all of the beta cells in your pancreas have been destroyed, and those that remain produce very little insulin. One of the great discoveries of 20th-century medicine was that externally produced insulin can substitute for the body's own missing or deficient supply. This exogenous insulin therapy can keep blood-glucose levels close enough to normal to maintain health.

Just because insulin therapy is effective, however, does not make it convenient. Nor can externally supplied insulin ever control blood sugar as well as normally produced insulin. Insulin cannot be taken by mouth: The body's digestive system would break it down and destroy it. For that reason, it must be injected or otherwise introduced directly into the bloodstream. Most people still inject their insulin, but researchers and manufacturers have developed more user-friendly ways to administer it, from the insulin jet to the insulin inhaler. Ask your health care team to advise you on the choice of a delivery device. Whatever method you choose, your health care providers will teach you how to take your insulin.

Previously, insulin was derived from beef or pork pancreas, but these types are no longer manufactured or sold in the United States. Most of the insulin used in the United States is now genetically engineered to be almost identical to human insulin.

Several different types of insulin are available; these are explained below. Each one is formulated to work at a certain speed, to deliver peak insulin at a certain time, and to last for a particular length of time. Your health care team will work with you to determine which insulin (or combination of insulins) works best for you and how often you need to administer it.

Types of Insulin

The Food and Drug Administration recognizes more than 20 types of insulin products. Each has a different time of onset, or when it begins acting; a different peak time, or when it is strongest; and a different duration of action, or how long it lasts. The type of insulin your health care provider prescribes for you depends in part on your blood-glucose levels and in part on your lifestyle. How often you take your insulin will hinge on the kind of insulin your doctor recommends.

Here are the five common insulin types:

1. Rapid-Acting Insulin:
lispro (Humalog®), aspart (Novolog®), glulisine (Apidra®)
- Onset: 5 to 15 minutes after injection
- Peak time: 60 to 90 minutes after injection
- Duration: 2 to 6 hours

2. Rapid-Acting Inhaled Insulin: Exubera®
- Onset: 5 to 10 minutes after use
- Peak time: about 60 minutes
- Duration: about 4 hours

3. Short-Acting Insulin: regular (Humulin R®, Novolin R®)
- Onset: within 30 minutes of injection
- Peak time: 2 to 3 hours after injection
- Duration: 3 to 8 hours

4. **Intermediate-Acting Insulin:**
NPH (Humulin N®, Novolin N®)
- Onset: 2 to 4 hours after injection
- Peak time: 4 to 12 hours after injection
- Duration: 12 to 18 hours

5. **Long-Acting Insulin: glargine (Lantus®), detemir (Levemir®)**
- Onset: 2 to 4 hours after injection
- No peak
- Duration: up to 24 hours (often less in children)

Insulin Pre-Mixes

Several manufacturers provide pre-mixed combinations of intermediate-acting insulin with either rapid- or short-acting insulin. These formulations include Novolog® 75/25, Humalog® 70/30, Humulin® 50/50, Humulin® 70/30, and Novolin® 70/30.

Many people, working with their health care team, combine different types of insulin for optimal control of their diabetes. All the types can be combined in one injection except the long-acting glargine or detemir, which must be taken separately.

Prescriptions

Laws vary from state to state and from country to country regarding whether or not you need a prescription for insulin or insulin syringes. Your health care provider and your pharmacist can tell you whether or not a prescription is required where you live. Even though prescriptions may not be required for obtaining insulin or syringes, many insurance companies require them for reimbursement purposes.

When to Take Insulin

People with type 2 diabetes may take insulin once a day or more. Most people with type 1 diabetes need to take insulin several times a day to manage their blood-glucose levels effectively.

Your health care provider will tell you when to take your insulin. In general, if you are on regular insulin alone or combined with a longer-acting insulin, you administer it 30 to 45 minutes before a meal. You take a rapid-acting insulin five to 10 minutes before you eat.

Once you and your health care provider arrive at an insulin plan that gives you the best control of your diabetes, you most likely won't be changing the type of insulin you take—at least for a while. You will still need to monitor your blood-glucose levels, however, as well as your sense of when your blood sugar may be too high or too low. And if your health care provider determines that you need to change your insulin plan, be prepared to monitor your blood glucose more often at first, and to make dosage adjustments in order to become stabilized on the new program. You may, however, need to change the amount or frequency of your insulin dose. Although people with type 2 diabetes rarely need to do so, many of them are taught to take supplemental insulin when their blood sugar goes above a certain level. Those with type 1 diabetes often take supplemental doses of regular insulin.

Key Information to Tell Your Doctor

Before you start taking insulin, your health care provider will ask you for a thorough medical history. Be sure to mention if you have any of the following conditions:

- Adrenal or pituitary gland problems
- Diarrhea
- Fever or infection
- Injury or trauma
- Kidney disease
- Nausea or vomiting
- Thyroid disease
- Recent surgery
- Any unusual or allergic reactions to other medicines, foods, dyes, or preservatives—and especially any known adverse reaction to insulin

You should also report all medications you are taking, including any nonprescription medicines, vitamins, nutritional supplements, or herbal products. Also tell your health care provider if you frequently drink caffeinated beverages or alcohol, if you smoke, or if you use recreational drugs. These may affect the way your insulin works. Check with your health care professional before stopping or starting any medication.

Using Injected Insulin

Your health care provider will show you how to give yourself insulin injections if this is the method you choose. You will learn to use a syringe or insulin pen, both of which have small needles that cause only the tiniest pricking sensation.

For information on how to use some of the newer insulin-delivery devices—including insulin inhalers, insulin pumps, and insulin injectors—see "Other Methods of Taking Insulin" on page 71.

The information given below about injecting insulin is intended as a reminder or convenient checklist. If you have any questions or are uncertain how to give yourself injections, contact a member of your health care team.

Locating Your Injections

Insulin can be injected into any fatty tissue under the skin, but it is most often injected into the outer thigh, the back of the hip (the "proximal buttocks," in physiologic lingo), and the lower abdomen, where it is absorbed best. Some people prefer to inject into their upper arms. To prevent irritation and other skin problems, change the injection site each time you give yourself insulin.

Here are some key points to keep in mind when deciding which injection site to use:

- Keep about 1 inch between sites.
- Leave at least 2 inches around your navel.
- Do not inject into broken or scarred skin. Do not inject into broken blood vessels.
- Try to inject your insulin at about the same time every day. Regular insulin alone or in combination with a longer-acting

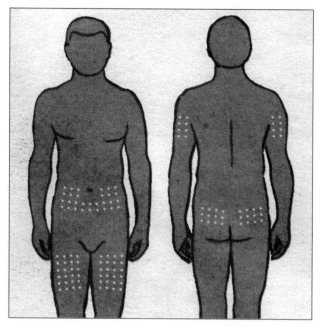

> Typical insulin-injection sites

insulin should be taken 30 to 45 minutes before meals; rapid-acting insulin should be taken five to 10 minutes before eating.

Getting Ready

Before you give yourself an injection, take the following steps:

• Wash your hands using soap and water; dry them thoroughly.

• Gather your supplies. You need a clean needle and syringe, insulin, alcohol wipes, and a sharps disposal container.

• Check that the medication is the type your doctor prescribed; that it has not expired; and that it is not discolored, frosted, or lumpy. If the medication does not look right to you, don't use it.

• Clean the insulin bottle. Wipe the rubber stopper with alcohol.

• Prepare the insulin. If you use cloudy-type insulin, roll the bottle or the pen device gently between your hands 10 to 20 times to redistribute the mixture evenly.

• Do not shake the container! Doing so deactivates the insulin.

Filling the Syringe

• Pull back the plunger until the end is even with the number of units of insulin you take; this brings air into the syringe.

• Insert the needle into the top of the bottle. Keep the bottle upright with the needle pointing straight in. Then push the plunger in all the way, adding air to the insulin bottle.

• Hold the bottle and syringe in one hand and turn your hand over so that the bottle is on top and the needle points up. Be sure the tip of the needle stays in the insulin.

• Pull back on the plunger again until the end of the plunger is about five units past the number of units of insulin you take. Look for any air bubbles in the insulin in the syringe. Tap the syringe to move any bubbles up, then push back on the plunger to force the bubbles and extra insulin back into the bottle. Stop when the end of the plunger is even with your precise dose.

• Remove the needle from the bottle.

• Don't be overly concerned about any small bubbles that remain in the syringe. They are not dangerous or harmful to you.

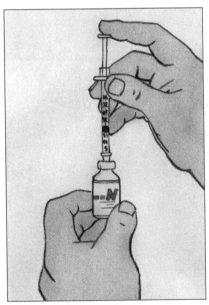

> Insert the needle into the bottle and push the plunger.

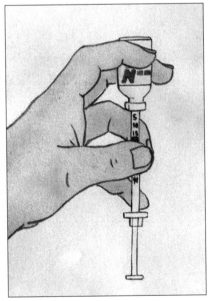

> Turn so that the bottle is on top.

Mixing Insulin

Your doctor may want you to take more than one kind of insulin. For example, you may need a combination of rapid- and longer-acting insulin to keep your blood glucose in the target range. Some people take mixed insulins one or two times a day and then shorter-acting insulin at other times of the day.

There are two ways to use mixed insulins. You can use a pre-mixed insulin, or you can mix the two types yourself. The pre-mixed insulin comes in fixed proportions of shorter- and longer-acting insulin and may not be right for everyone. Mixing the two types of insulin yourself allows greater customizing of the insulin program.

If you do mix insulins, both types can usually be put into the syringe at the same time, allowing you to take one injection rather than two. Check with your doctor or pharmacist as to whether your insulins can be mixed. Follow these steps for combining insulins into one injection:

- Clean the tops of both vials with an alcohol swab.
- Inject air into the longer-acting (cloudy) insulin vial in the same amount as you will draw out in the later steps. Do not pull insulin into the syringe.
- Take the needle and syringe out of the vial.
- Using the same needle and syringe, inject air into the rapid-acting (clear) insulin vial in the same amount as you will draw out.
- Turn the vial and syringe upside down—that is, with the needle pointing up. Make sure the tip of the needle stays in the liquid insulin.
- Hold the vial and syringe with one hand.
- Use the other hand to pull back the plunger until slightly more than the required dose of rapid-acting insulin is in the syringe.
- Remove any large air bubbles: With the needle still pointing up, carefully expel the bubbles by pushing up on the plunger, being careful not to expel too much of the insulin. Check that the in-sulin in the syringe is the right amount.
- Remove the needle and syringe from the vial.

Next, move to the other vial of insulin.

- Gently roll between your palms at least 10 to 20 times the vial of longer-acting insulin.
- Insert the needle into the vial of longer-acting insulin.
- Turn the vial and syringe upside down—that is, with the needle pointing up. Make sure the tip of the needle stays in the liquid insulin.
- Hold the vial and syringe with one hand.
- Use the other hand to pull back on the plunger until you have added to the rapid-acting insulin already in the syringe the amount of longer-acting insulin prescribed by your doctor. (You should end up with the plunger on the mark denoting the total of the combination of rapid- and longer-acting insulin.)
- Be careful not to push any of the rapid-acting insulin into the longer-acting vial.
- Remove the needle and syringe from the vial.

Don't worry if you forget to put air in the vial a few times. However, eventually a vacuum will be created in the vial, keeping you from drawing out the insulin. This suction may even draw any insulin already in the syringe into the vial. You can correct this by injecting air several times with a syringe into a vial to relieve the vacuum.

Injecting the Insulin

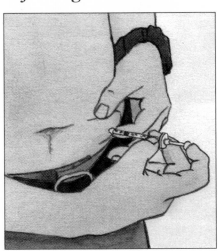

- Clean the injection site by rubbing it with an alcohol wipe.
- Gently pull up and pinch about 1 inch of skin. Do not squeeze hard.
- Hold the needle and syringe at right angles to the skin. Insert the needle into the pinched skin, pushing it in all the way to its base.

- Push in the plunger. Press until the syringe is empty.
- Let go of the skin, then withdraw the needle.
- Don't rub the site after you remove the needle; if there is any blood, gently wipe it away, place the alcohol swab over the site, and maintain gentle pressure for 30 seconds.

Disposing of the Needle and Syringe

- After you inject, put the needle and syringe directly into a sharps disposal container. Never lay them down anywhere. If you don't use a sharps container, be sure to put the cap back on the needle before you discard it.
- When the sharps container is full, put it into a garbage bag and secure the top. Label the bag "needles."
- Call your local waste company to ask about disposal requirements for needles. You can also call the Coalition for Safe Community Needle Disposal at 800-643-1643.

Using Injection Pens

Some people who take insulin find it more convenient to use injection pens, which can carry multiple accurate doses and are more discreet than syringes. There are two types: disposable and nondisposable.

A disposable pen comes filled with insulin and is used multiple times. When it is empty, you throw the pen away. With nondisposable pens, you replace the medication cartridge when it is empty.

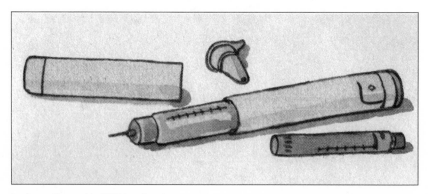

> A nondisposable (CK) insulin pen

The pens can use a single type of insulin or they can use a mixture prepared by the manufacturer. Both types of pens require a pen needle, which is screwed onto the tip of the pen before injection. Pen needles come in various lengths and thicknesses. Your diabetes educator or health care provider can help you decide on the right size and will show you how to use the pen. Always review the instructions enclosed with your pen. Follow the general guidelines below.

Preparing the pen

- Wash and dry your hands thoroughly.
- Remove the pen cap.
- Check the medication to verify that it is the type your doctor prescribed; that it hasn't expired; and that it's not discolored, frosted, or lumpy. If the medication doesn't look right to you, don't use it; get a new cartridge or a new disposable pen.
- Attach a needle to the pen according to the directions that came with the pen. Don't leave a used needle attached to the pen.
- Mix the drug by rolling the pen between the palms of your hands about 20 times; you can also tip the pen back and forth.

Priming the pen and setting the dose

- Dial the pen to deliver two or three units of medication.
- Hold the pen with the needle pointing up.
- Tap the barrel of the pen. This will ensure that any air bubbles in the cartridge float to the top.
- Prime your pen to ensure that it's working with a trial "air shot": Push down firmly on the pen's injector button to "shoot" medication into the air. You should see a couple of drops of medication come out of the needle. If nothing comes out, try doing another air shot. If medication still doesn't come out, your pen may be low on medication or the needle may not be connected properly. Refer to the troubleshooting tips in the directions that came with the pen.
- Set your dose. Dial the pen to deliver the amount of insulin you need to take. As you turn the dial, you should hear a clicking sound. Your pen is now ready to use.

Inject the insulin
- Clean the injection site with an alcohol swab.
- Pinch up a fold of skin surrounding the site you've selected. Hold it firmly with one hand.
- In the other hand, hold the injection pen like a pencil.
- Insert the needle straight into the pinched-up skin. Thin adults or children may need to inject at a 45° angle. Make sure the needle gets all the way into the fatty tissue below the skin.
- Push the pen injection button. Unless you take a very small dose, the injection should take a couple of seconds.
- Let go of the skin, then withdraw the needle.
- Don't rub the site after you remove the needle; if there is any blood, gently wipe it away, place the alcohol swab over the site, and maintain gentle pressure for 30 seconds.

After the injection
- Remove the needle by unscrewing it.
- Follow the instructions under "Disposing of the Needle and Syringe," page 66.

If You Miss a Dose
Do your best never to miss any of your insulin injections. If you do miss the time for a dose, take it as soon as you can after that. However, if it is almost time for your next dose, take only that dose; do not take double doses. Check your blood sugar and take whatever action you have been taught to take if your blood sugar is too high (or too low). Know the signs of low and high blood sugar, and make sure a close family member or friend can recognize these signs as well. Contact your health care provider at once if you have any problems.

What to Watch for If You're Taking Insulin
Keep these precautions in mind if you take insulin:

- To reduce the chance of high or low blood-sugar levels, space your meals and insulin injections properly. Whenever you are uncertain about your blood sugar, use a glucose meter to check your levels.

• Try not to change the brand and type of insulin syringe unless your health care provider tells you to. Use a syringe only once; throw away both syringe and needle in a sharps container or other closed receptacle to prevent accidental needle sticks. If a special container isn't available, be sure the needle is capped.

• Wear a medical alert bracelet or necklace. Alternatively, carry an identification card displaying your name and address, condition, medication, and health care provider's name and phone number.

• If you develop a cold, diarrhea, vomiting, or any acute infection or illness, contact your health care provider immediately and increase your frequency of blood sugar checks. You may need to adjust your insulin dose or take other steps, but don't stop taking your insulin. Ask your health care provider in advance what you should do if you become ill.

• If you are a longtime smoker and suddenly stop, you may need to change your insulin dose. Smoking increases your body's resistance to insulin. Before you quit, tell your health care provider in case it is necessary to adjust your insulin dose.

• Many nonprescription cough and cold products contain sugar. These can affect diabetes control. Avoid products that contain sugar, and talk to your practitioner before you take any over-the-counter medication.

• If you are going to have surgery, inform your surgeon well ahead of time that you take insulin. Your surgeon will then tell you (likewise in advance) what you should do with your insulin dose on the day of your surgery.

Possible Side Effects

Learn how and when you should monitor your blood sugar and what steps to take if high or low blood sugar occurs. Be alert to the symptoms of hypoglycemia and hyperglycemia.

Hypoglycemia

People who take insulin need to be particularly alert to the symptoms of hypoglycemia (low blood glucose). Symptoms of hypoglycemia include feeling shaky, breaking out in a sweat, hunger, nervousness, dizziness, weakness, and confusion. Left unchecked, hypoglycemia may cause you to lose track of your actions or surroundings or to lose consciousness. Let others know what to do in the event of a severe reaction—one where you may be unable to take care of yourself. (See the box on page 43 for a list of the symptoms of hypoglycemia. In addition, chapter 10 explains hypoglycemia in detail—notably the need to treat it promptly.)

Hyperglycemia

Symptoms of high blood sugar (hyperglycemia) develop much more slowly than those of low blood sugar. They include dizziness, dry mouth, flushed or dry skin, a fruity breath odor, loss of appetite, nausea, stomachache, unusual thirst, and frequent urination. Extremely high blood-glucose levels can lead to diabetic ketoacidosis (DKA), a condition that can lead to a coma if it is not treated. (Chapter 3 discusses this condition in detail.)

When to Call Your Health Care Provider

Call your health care provider right away if you experience any of the following:

- Problems that prevent you from giving yourself an injection
- Accidental injection of a wrong dose
- Injection of medication in the wrong area
- Rash, redness, or swelling at the injection site
- Fever
- Any signs of an allergic reaction, such as trouble breathing, hives, or a rash anywhere on the body
- Blood-glucose levels that are frequently too low or too high
- Bleeding from the injection site for more than 10 minutes
- Pain at the injection site that does not go away

Storing Your Insulin

Store insulin according to the manufacturer's instructions. Never freeze insulin or let it get above 86° F. Throw away any unused insulin after the expiration date, or 28 days after opening it.

In general, you can store insulin at room temperature or in the refrigerator. Keep unopened insulin in your refrigerator. Insulin degrades and becomes useless if it gets too hot or too cold. Never put insulin in the freezer or leave it in a hot car or on a sunny windowsill. Once you start using a bottle, you can keep it at room temperature, but avoid keeping it in places likely to become very warm, such as your car. Write on the label the date that is one month away after opening; after that date, dispose of any unused portion. Pen-injector cartridges may be kept at room temperature (approximately 77° F or cooler) for up to 10 days. Read the manufacturer's instructions; different pens have different storage instructions.

You should keep on hand an extra bottle of each type of insulin you use in case you run out. Keep these spare bottles in the refrigerator.

When you travel, put all of your supplies in an insulated bag and keep the bag with you. Additionally, always carry a prescription for needles and syringes with you when you travel in case you visit a state or country that requires one. This will come in handy if you need to buy more or in the event you are questioned about the syringes at Customs. Never put your supplies in luggage that you check through.

As with any other medications, keep your insulin out of the reach of children.

Other Methods of Taking Insulin

Although injection is the most common and most economical way to take insulin, you may want to consider some newer methods and discuss them with your health care team. Cost may be an issue with the methods described below, so be sure to check with your insurance company to see whether the methods included here are covered completely, in part, or not at all.

Insulin Injectors

An insulin injector uses a high-pressure propulsion system to shoot a fine spray of insulin through your skin. Some people find injectors to be less painful than needle injections. And there's an added advantage: They spread the insulin over a wider area than an injection does, so the insulin enters your bloodstream faster.

Injector use is not widespread, perhaps because the devices are bulky and inconvenient to carry. Also, many people have trouble adjusting the spray so that it penetrates the skin with minimal discomfort. Insulin injectors are expensive, and most insurance plans do not cover them.

Inhaled Insulin

In January 2006, the Food and Drug Administration approved a new form of insulin that can be inhaled. Now available by prescription, human-inhaled insulin powder (brand name Exubera®) offers a breakthrough in ease of use for at least one form of insulin therapy.

Insulin inhalers deliver the rapid-acting insulin that you take right before meals. You breathe a powder-like form of the drug into your lungs, where it is absorbed quickly into the bloodstream. You may still need to take long-acting insulin by injection, but you can avoid the inconvenience of having to give yourself an injection every time you have a meal.

Inhaled insulin can cause coughing, shortness of breath, sore throat, dry mouth, and irritation to the nasal passages. People who smoke or who have quit smoking within the last six months should not use inhaled insulin, nor is it recommended for people with asthma, bronchitis, or emphysema. If you use inhaled insulin, your health care provider will need to perform a lung-function test before and six months after you start taking it, then once a year after that to make certain that there has been no diminution in lung function.

Insurance reimbursement may be an issue for some users. Check first with your health insurance company to make sure it covers inhaled insulin.

Insulin Pumps

For people who have struggled to control their diabetes or who need tighter regulation of their blood-glucose levels, insulin pumps may be the answer. They are also a good choice for those looking for a more convenient way to get their insulin.

Insulin pumps deliver precise doses of rapid-acting insulin through a flexible plastic tube called a catheter. They deliver both a constant infusion (called the basal rate) and additional doses as needed (called boluses). The pump itself is a small device about the size of a deck of cards; it is worn on a belt or carried in a pocket. Computerized components in the pump regulate how much insulin is released at different times of the day. The catheter is inserted with a small needle, but the needle is then removed, leaving only the tiny plastic catheter end in the skin. To reduce the risk of infection, the user moves the insertion site to a new location every few days. Some pumps now have sensors as well that measure your blood-sugar level every few minutes and transmit the result to the pump. That sensor uses a separate catheter that is placed under the skin and changed every few days.

Of all the artificial insulin-delivery devices, insulin pumps come the closest to replicating the natural functioning of the pancreas. This makes them highly effective at keeping blood-glucose levels normal throughout the day. The steady insulin supply released by the pump helps avoid

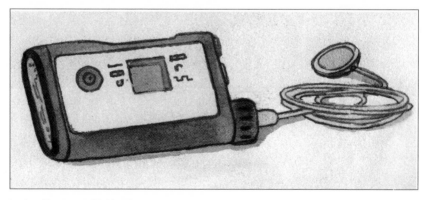

> Insulin pump with blood-sugar sensor

the peaks and valleys of insulin levels in the bloodstream that can plague people who inject their insulin at several fixed intervals a day.

Over time, an insulin pump may allow you to follow a more flexible eating schedule and enable you to exercise longer and more intensely. It may also be the best solution if you have a variable work schedule that makes it difficult to adhere to a regular pattern of injections.

Bear in mind that insulin pumps do not free you from the necessity of monitoring your blood-glucose levels regularly. Even the ones with sensors require calibration at least twice a day. Currently, pumps require you to specify how much insulin the device should administer before each meal.

Expense is one big drawback. Most insulin pumps cost about $5,000 to $7,000, and the supplies can run an additional $1,500 a year. Check with your insurance company to see what percentage of the pump and supplies it will cover—and, as always, discuss the option fully with your health care provider.

Looking to the Future

Medical researchers are constantly looking for better and more convenient ways to control diabetes with insulin. One new system being developed is a "transdermal" patch that would work much the same way as a nicotine patch, delivering doses directly through the skin. Another technique under study involves a form of insulin called buccal insulin, which would be sprayed into the back of the throat; there it would be readily absorbed into the bloodstream, avoiding some of the potential complications of inhaled insulin. And scientists continue to explore the possibility of an insulin pill that would be impervious to attack by the body's digestive system.

Common to all these approaches is an attempt to make insulin delivery both more convenient and more akin to the body's natural process for regulating blood glucose. The ultimate goal is a system that provides the best management of diabetes with the least effort and inconvenience on the part of the individual.

6 Medications for Type 2 Diabetes

For people with type 2 diabetes, the mainstay of contemporary treatment is a blend of diet and exercise, often combined with oral medications and sometimes insulin.

Diet and Exercise Alone May Work

Through a combination of careful meal planning and regular exercise, some people with type 2 diabetes are able to keep their blood glucose at normal levels. Good control may be permanent or last several years. Other people need medication from the start. Even those who are able to control their blood glucose at first without taking any medicine may eventually require medications to manage their diabetes. For still others, the amount of insulin the pancreas makes, even when stimulated with medications, remains very low. These people often need to take insulin. Sometimes, they take both oral medications and supplemental insulin.

Medication for Type 2 Diabetes

If you have type 2 diabetes, your body is usually resistant to insulin and does not produce enough of this metabolic hormone. For decades, the only medication available to treat type 2 diabetes was a type of drug called a sulfonylurea, which increases insulin production. Nowadays, by contrast, several other drug types are available to treat insulin resistance and production, as well as other aspects of high blood-glucose levels. This wide range of medicines enables your doctor to tailor your diabetes medication to your specific needs as those needs change.

Commonly Prescribed Medications

The medications most commonly prescribed for type 2 diabetes are explained below. Most are taken by mouth in pill form. The list is organized by drug class and includes side effects whenever they are known. The examples are given as generic drug name first, followed by the various brand names in parentheses.

Sulfonylureas
[Examples: glipizide (Glucotrol®, Glucotrol XL®); glimepiride (Amaryl®); glyburide (DiaBeta®, Micronase®]
These drugs stimulate the pancreas to make more insulin. Because these drugs increase insulin release, they can cause low blood sugar (hypoglycemia) as a side effect.

Meglitinides
[Examples: repaglanide (Prandin®); nateglinide (Starlix®)]
These drugs act quickly to stimulate your pancreas to make more insulin. They tend to work soon after being administered and so are more effective than some other drugs at preventing blood-sugar spikes after meals. Because these drugs increase insulin release, they can cause low blood sugar (hypoglycemia) as a side effect.

Thiazolidinediones (TZD)
[Examples: pioglitazone (Actos®); rosiglitazone (Avandia®)]
These drugs increase insulin sensitivity and lower blood glucose without increasing in-sulin production. They work by making the amount of insulin in your body more effective. (They may be taken alone or in combination with other drugs.) The medications can cause fluid retention, so let your doctor know if you start gaining weight. Because they do not increase insulin production, they do not usually cause low blood sugar (hypoglycemia).

> At press time, the FDA was reviewing clinical trial data showing increased risk of heart-related incidents in patients taking Avandia®.

People with type 2 diabetes are often started on a certain medication; then, if it becomes clear that their therapy goals are not being met, a second medication may be added from a different drug category. Most health care providers would rather add than switch medication, because drug classes act in different ways—and the effects are cumulative.

In some cases, if a person has complications related to diabetes or a serious illness such as an infection, insulin will be used to start treatment because it is reliable and takes effect rapidly. Once the person's health improves, however, he or she may be able to give up insulin and take pills instead.

Biguanides
[Examples: metformin (Glucophage®, Fortamet®)]
These drugs block the release of glucose by the liver and reduce the body's resistance to insulin. They lower blood-glucose levels without increasing insulin production, and that makes them less likely than some drugs to cause low blood sugar (hypoglycemia). If you have kidney disease, however, these medications may not be right for you. They can cause diarrhea initially, which usually resolves.

Alpha-glucosidase (AG) inhibitors
[Examples: acarbase (Precose®); miglitol (Glyset®)]
These medications block the absorption of carbohydrates from your digestive tract, lowering post-meal glucose levels. Common side effects include excess gas, abdominal discomfort, and diarrhea.

Incretin mimetic
[Example: exenatide (Byetta®)]
This new drug helps people with type 2 diabetes who cannot manage their diabetes using oral medications. Given by injection twice daily, it enhances insulin secretion and suppresses the body's production of glucose. As an added benefit, it slows the rate at which food empties from

the stomach, thereby reducing appetite. Exenatide is approved as an additional treatment for people who already take metformin, a sulfonylurea, a thiazolidinedione, or a combination of these drugs. Nausea is a significant side effect, but in time it usually dissipates. Another drug, sitagliptin (Januvia®), is available as a pill and works in similar fashion to exenatide (Byetta®) but is not as effective in weight loss.

Amylino mimetic
[Example: pramlintide (Symlin®)]
This synthetic hormone resembles amylin, a human hormone secreted along with insulin by the pancreas after meals that helps regulate blood glucose. Pramlintide is used in addition to insulin for treating type 2 and type 1 diabetes in people who cannot control their diabetes with insulin alone. Generally, the insulin dose is reduced by about 50 percent when you begin taking pramlintide (your doctor may increase it later, depending on your blood-glucose levels). The drug is taken by injection before meals; nausea can be a side effect.

Insulin Pre-Mixes
Several pills combine two different diabetes medications in a single tablet, simplifying the dosing process. Combinations currently available include: glipizide and metformin (Metaglip®); glyburide and metformin (Glucovance®); rosiglitazone and metformin (Avandamet®); pioglitazone and metformin (Actoplus Met®); and rosiglitazone and glimepiride (Avandaryl®), and Janumet® (sitagliptin and metformin).

Insulin for Type 2 Diabetes
No matter how hard some people work to manage their disease with exercise, diet, and oral medications, their blood-glucose levels continue to climb above the normal range too often. The deterioration may result from reduced insulin production, increased insulin resistance, or a combination of the two. When this happens, insulin must be used to control the diabetes. Sometimes, doctors add insulin to oral medications; other times they stop some or all of the oral medications and continue with insulin alone.

Taking insulin for type 2 diabetes is not as complicated as it is for type 1. Rather than taking several injections or doses a day, you might take insulin only once or twice. These doses may be combinations of different types of insulin or a single type. Nor is it necessary for those with type 2 to monitor blood glucose as often—once they have the disease under control, that is. Work with your health care provider to determine the best plan for insulin and glucose monitoring.

Some Precautions If You Take Diabetes Medications

Here are some points to keep in mind if you take diabetes medications:

• Diabetes medicines never take the place of healthy eating and exercise. Continue to follow your meal plan and exercise regimen according to your doctor's guidance.

• Review your blood-glucose levels with your doctor. She or he will tell you what the best range is for you. If your monitoring reveals that your levels have begun falling low or climbing high, call your doctor and discuss what to do.

• You may need to take your medications even when you are sick. (Check this with your doctor.) If you are too ill to follow your regular diet, check your blood sugar often and follow the dietary lessons you have learned. If you are unable to eat much, call your doctor. He or she may need to adjust your medication (never attempt this yourself unless you have been taught what to do as part of a sick-day plan!). If you take insulin, adjust your doses according to the sick-day plan provided by your health care team.

7 Meal Planning to Manage Diabetes

Good eating habits are important for everyone, but they're crucial if you have diabetes. By learning how different foods affect your body—and by using that knowledge to change your eating habits—you can manage your diabetes more effectively and reduce the risk of complications.

As you know by now, diabetes impairs the body's ability to metabolize glucose. Untreated, it causes blood-glucose levels to rise. High blood-glucose levels lead to many short-term problems, such as fatigue, weakness, frequency of urination, blurred vision, dehydration, blood-chemistry imbalance, and confusion. Long-term problems—those that develop after a year or more of poorly controlled diabetes—include heart and kidney disease, circulatory problems, nerve damage, vision loss, and sexual dysfunction.

Meal planning is a key component of diabetes management because it enables you, at least in part, to control your blood-glucose levels from the "outside"—that is, through food choices and the timing of meals and snacks. In effect, your own voluntary diet choices can replace the involuntary, "internal" controls that diabetes has compromised.

Does this mean you must give up all the foods you like? Or that meals will no longer be enjoyable? Far from it. It does mean, however, that you need to think more carefully about what you're eating, and that your top priority in planning meals and selecting snacks must always be how the foods you choose will affect your blood glucose.

Meal Planning and Your Diabetes Type

If you have type 2 diabetes, you face different dietary issues than people with type 1. Because this form of the disease often traces to obesity and being overweight, weight loss and maintaining a good weight are customary cornerstones of the dietary approach to managing the condition. In fact, losing as little as 5 to 7 percent of your current body weight (and keeping that weight off) can lower your blood-glucose levels to the point where you may be able to reduce the amount of diabetes medication you take. Many people will benefit from losing even more weight.

If you have type 2 diabetes and are being treated with insulin, it's important that you coordinate your diet and insulin program. If you have type 1 diabetes, you must coordinate your diet with your insulin program for the simple reason that how much carbohydrate you eat determines how much insulin your body requires.

Until recently, the conventional wisdom was to plan meals around fixed insulin doses and schedules. No longer. Now the recommended approach is to tailor insulin injections to eating habits. But that doesn't translate into "Anything goes" as far as dietary choices are concerned. With both type 2 and type 1 diabetes, a consistent pattern of eating balanced meals on a regular schedule—complemented by frequent monitoring of blood sugar to determine precise insulin doses—is vital to controlling blood-glucose levels.

Understanding What You Eat

For both types of diabetes, eating the right combination of proteins, carbohydrates, and fats can help keep your blood-sugar levels closer to normal. People with diabetes are at increased risk of heart disease, so it likewise makes good sense to choose a heart-healthy diet that is low in fat and high in fiber.

How do you decide what to eat and how much? Start by understanding what you eat. Talk to the dietitian on your health care team about types of food and their effects on your body, with special focus on portion sizes and what exactly is appropriate and inappropriate for you. But you should also educate yourself and learn all you can about different foods and how they affect your blood-glucose levels.

Food groups

Understanding good nutrition begins with knowing about the three main food groups—carbohydrates, fats, and proteins. It's also smart to learn about the different types of carbohydrates and fats, which can have radically different effects on health. If you are overweight, eating fewer calories and exercising more will help you reduce your weight.

Carbohydrates

Carbohydrates are the main source of fuel for the body. They raise levels of blood glucose, which cells "burn" for energy. There are three basic groups of carbohydrates: sugars, starches, and fiber.

Sugars

Also known as simple carbohydrates, sugars occur naturally in foods such as fruit, milk, honey, and some vegetables. Refined, or processed, sugars can also be added to many kinds of foods, from cereals and yogurt to candy and desserts. The body readily converts most sugars into blood glucose, so all sugars can raise blood-glucose levels quickly.

Starches

Starches—a type of complex carbohydrate—are found in breads, bagels, rice, beans, cereals, pasta, and dried beans, as well as in corn, peas, potatoes, sweet potatoes, and winter squash (acorn, Hubbard, butternut, and pumpkin). Even though starches, like sugars, are ultimately converted into glucose, the body digests starches more slowly than sugars. Starches therefore raise blood-sugar levels less quickly than sugars.

Fiber

Foods such as vegetables, fruits, and whole grains contain fiber, which is a form of complex carbohydrate the body cannot digest or absorb. Most fiber doesn't raise blood-sugar levels; in fact, because of its ability to slow the passage of food through the stomach and intestines, it can help keep blood-glucose levels from rising too quickly. Increasing the amount of fiber in the diet can also improve blood-cholesterol levels. Some fibers, however, are absorbed and can elevate your blood glucose.

Fat

Fat is a source of energy and plays other beneficial roles. It supplies calories without raising blood-glucose levels. Sometimes the body uses fat immediately for energy, but it also readily stores it away—one of the reasons fat can increase your weight. Saturated fats can also raise blood-cholesterol levels and thus increase the risk of heart disease. Fat is a calorie-dense food: It packs nine calories per gram as opposed to four per gram for proteins and carbohydrates, which accounts for its tendency to cause weight gain. As explained below, some types of fat are healthier than others—and some are decidedly unhealthy.

Healthy fats. Monounsaturated fats are good for your heart because they lower "bad" low-density lipoprotein (LDL) cholesterol levels and raise the levels of "good" high-density lipoprotein (HDL) cholesterol. The chief sources of monounsaturated fats are certain vegetable oils, including olive, canola, and peanut oils. Avocados and some nuts contain these fats as well.

Polyunsaturated fats also lower LDL cholesterol levels in your blood and are good for your heart. (As an added benefit, they may raise HDL cholesterol; the scientific jury is still out on the issue.) Vegetable oils such as corn, safflower, and soybean oil contain high levels of polyunsaturated fats, as do some seeds, nuts, and fish. But plan carefully: These fats still contain lots of calories.

Unhealthy fats. Animal products such as meat, poultry, milk, lard, and butter contain saturated fats. These fats raise LDL cholesterol levels and are not good for the heart. Coconut and palm oils also contain high levels of saturated fat.

Adding hydrogen to vegetable oils—a process known as hydrogenation or partial hydrogenation—makes them more solid, which can enhance palatability and retard spoilage. But it also turns these oils into trans fats, which raise levels of LDL cholesterol without raising HDL cholesterol and therefore promote the buildup of atherosclerotic plaques in blood vessels. Many processed foods contain these fats.

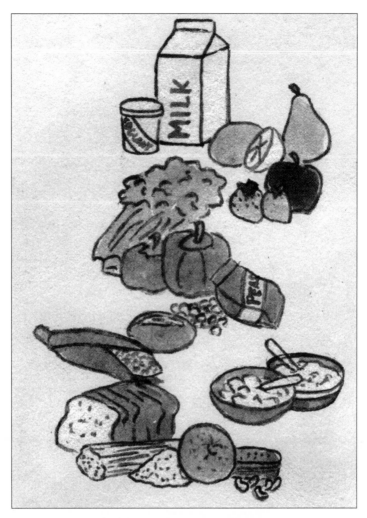

> Many different food types contain carbohydrates.

Protein

Protein helps the body build and repair muscle and other tissues and provides a slow and sustained source of energy. It has little or no effect on blood-sugar levels. However, many foods that contain protein also contain saturated fat; for example, many meats as well as dairy products made from milk contain fat. Choosing low-fat proteins such as fish

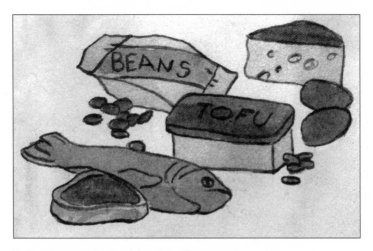

> Protein comes from a rich variety of sources.

and certain vegetables gives you the benefits of protein without the extra calories and other health negatives of saturated fat.

Plant protein. Fresh and dried beans, peas, and other legumes; nuts; and soy products such as tofu and soy milk contain plant protein. These sources tend to be cholesterol-free and low in saturated fat.

Animal protein. Meat, poultry, fish, cheese, milk, and eggs contain animal protein. This type of protein can be high in saturated fat and cholesterol, so choose forms that are lower in fat, such as lean cuts of beef, white-meat turkey, or chicken without skin, and low-fat versions of dairy products.

How to Make a Healthy Meal Plan

For people with diabetes, there are many ways to plan healthy meals. Two common methods are carbohydrate counting and food exchanges. For those who need to lose weight, it may be necessary to count calories as well. Work with your health care team to find the method (or mix of methods) that works best for you. Your team will also instruct you about how to time meals and check your blood-sugar levels.

Meal plan for: _____ Date: _____

Notes:
_____
_____
_____

Healthcare provider: _____ Phone: _____
_____

Meal	Number of Exchanges/Choices	Total Carbs	Menu Ideas
MEAL #1 Time ____	____ Carbohydrate Group ____ Starch ____ Fruit ____ Milk ____ ____ Vegetables ____ Fat Group _____ ____ Meat Group _____		
SNACK Time ____	___ _____ ___ _____		
MEAL #2 Time ____	____ Carbohydrate Group ____ Starch ____ Fruit ____ Milk ____ ____ Vegetables ____ Fat Group _____ ____ Meat Group _____		
SNACK Time ____	___ _____ ___ _____		
MEAL #3 Time ____	____ Carbohydrate Group ____ Starch ____ Fruit ____ Milk ____ ____ Vegetables ____ Fat Group _____ ____ Meat Group _____		
SNACK Time ____	___ _____ ___ _____		

> With your health care provider's assistance, fill in this form for planning meals. If you have a favorite food, be sure to mention it. There are ways to include all kinds of foods. If weight loss is a goal for you, be sure to mention that as well.

Counting Carbs

Carbohydrate counting means keeping track of the total amount of carbohydrates you eat at each meal or snack and staying within the limits you and your health care provider have determined are right for you. This method is particularly valuable if you take insulin or other diabetes medications and must monitor your blood-sugar levels meal by meal.

You can use food labels to count grams of carbohydrates. For foods that lack nutrition labels (such as fresh fruits, vegetables, and meats and other unpackaged foods), you can consult books and other sources of information that list their carbohydrate content.

Food Exchanges

Food exchanges are another popular way to make food choices within a healthy meal plan. Once you've established targets or limits with your health care team, you can "exchange" one food for another so long as you stay within a group of foods that have similar amounts of carbohydrates, protein, fat, and calories. Using food exchanges works well with unlabeled foods.

Calories

The American Diabetes Association suggests that overweight people with diabetes moderately restrict calories. With your dietitian, determine how many calories you need each day to maintain your weight. Now subtract 250 from that number and confine your daily caloric intake to the result; you will shed a little more than half a pound every 10 days. (One pound of fat contains about 4,000 calories.) Cutting calories like this plus exercising should allow you to lose even more.

Timing Meals

There are two important points about timing your meals. First, it is better to eat small meals more often than big meals less often. This pattern requires less insulin and helps you lose weight. Second, when you eat at the same times every day, you set a pattern that helps keep your blood-sugar level within good limits. Here are some tips for developing healthy meal patterns:

- Spread the carbohydrates you eat throughout the day. Try to eat more carbohydrates when you are physically active.
- Establish an appropriate amount of carbohydrates for each meal and snack you eat, and stick to that quantity every day.
- Eat several smaller meals a day rather than two or three larger meals.
- Do not skip meals.

Checking Your Blood Sugar

Some people with diabetes—especially those with type 1 diabetes and those with type 2 who take insulin or other diabetes medications—monitor their blood-sugar levels regularly, several times a day. Even if you won't eventually have to be quite so rigorous, it helps to monitor your level at different times of the day as you begin your new diet so that you can see how different foods affect your blood sugar. This is the best way to determine whether a certain food might be appropriate or not in your diet. For example, if your blood-glucose level is high two to three hours after you eat a given food, you should reduce the portion of that food in the future. If, by contrast, your glucose is at a reasonable level after you eat a certain food, you can be reasonably sure that you are practicing wise portion control.

Your health care provider will work with you to explain how often and when to check your blood glucose and what your target ranges should be at different times of the day (see chapter 4).

Balance Your Meals

Talk to your health care provider to learn how to balance your meals and how much of each food type to eat. Healthy eating means consuming a variety of foods. Try to plan your meals around whole grains, vegetables, and fruits. Limit meat and other fatty foods. You can use the plate model shown on page 91 as a guide.

Measure the Foods You Eat

There is more to a healthy diet than eating the right foods: You must also eat the right amount of the right foods. That means learning about serving sizes.

Even though people routinely interchange the terms, a portion is not the same thing as a serving. A portion is a helping—any amount of one type of food you put on your plate. Portions can thus be large or small. A serving, on the other hand, is a measured, fixed amount of food.

The trick with servings is that they vary from food to food. In planning your meals and tracking what you eat, you need to know how much of a given food equals a single serving. With packaged foods, that's easy: You simply read the label. With other foods such as meats and fresh vegetables, you must do more research; you may need to measure until you know what one serving looks like.

How to measure

You can measure your food with measuring spoons and cups, and you can weigh it on a scale. Many people with diabetes use a small postage scale to measure what they eat. Your health care provider will help you learn how to measure a serving.

Using a scale or measuring cups is a sure way of knowing how much you're eating. But what if you're at a dinner party or in a restaurant where you're unfamiliar with what one serving of a particular dish looks like? Here are some easy rules of thumb to help you balance your meal without measuring:

- Cover one-fourth of your plate with grains or other starches (potatoes, pasta, rice, peas, corn).
- Cover one-fourth of the plate with protein (meat, poultry, fish, tofu).
- Cover half your plate with vegetables that are nonstarchy (broccoli, cucumbers, lettuce, tomatoes, cauliflower).

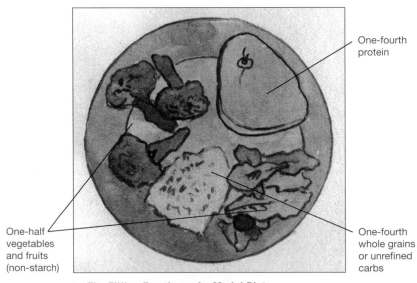

One-fourth protein

One-half vegetables and fruits (non-starch)

One-fourth whole grains or unrefined carbs

> The Filling Fractions of a Model Plate

1 TEASPOON
The tip of the thumb or a penny

1 TABLESPOON
A thumb, from the knuckle, or a quarter

1/2 CUP
A cupped hand or a golf ball

1 CUP
A fist or a tennis ball

2 TO 3 OUNCES
A small palm or a deck of cards

Read the Label

Federal law requires all packaged food sold in the United States to carry a label indicating the amount of fat, protein, and carbohydrate per serving, and to specify how many servings are in the package. The nutrition label also lists how much of each type of fat and carbohydrate the food contains, how much salt and cholesterol, and how much of any vitamins and minerals.

The food label helps you in three key ways:

1. It tells you how many grams of carbohydrates are in a serving—particularly helpful if you're counting carbohydrates. Pay attention to what the package defines as a serving size (it might be smaller than what you had in mind).

Nutrition Facts

Serving Size 1 cup
Servings Per Container 2

Amount Per Serving

Calories 93   Calories from Fat 20

	% Daily Value*
Total Fat 2g	**3%**
Saturated Fat 2g **3%**	
Trans Fat 0g	
Cholesterol 10mg	**3%**
Sodium 890mg	**37%**
Total Carbohydrate 13g	**4%**
Dietary Fiber 1g	**4%**
Sugars 1g	
Protein 6g	

Vitamin A 4%	•	Vitamin C 2%
Calcium 15%	•	Iron 4%

*Percent Daily Values are based on a 2,000 calorie diet. Your Daily Values may be higher or lower depending on your calorie needs.

Calories. To help maintain a healthy weight, look for foods low in calories.

Total Fat. This number tells you the total amount of fat in each serving. Limit fats, especially if you are trying to lose some weight.

Saturated Fat. Look for foods with little or no saturated fat. Saturated fat raises cholesterol, which can increase your risk of heart disease.

Trans Fat. This number tells you if the food includes trans fat. Trans fat is bad for your heart. Try to avoid food containing trans fat.

Total Carbohydrate. This number tells you how many carbs are in each serving. If you are carb counting, this number will help you fit the food into your meal plan.

Dietary Fiber. This number tells you how much of the carbohydrate in the food is fiber. Fiber is a good kind of carbohydrate. So look for foods containing fiber to add to your meal plan.

Serving Size. This number tells you how much of the food makes up a single serving. If you eat more of the food than this amount, the other numbers, like the amount of fat and carbs, will also increase.

Sugars. This number includes both natural and added sugars. Your dietitian can help you figure out how much sugar is okay for you to eat.

Protein. This states the total amount of protein in a serving of the food.

2. It helps you figure out how many servings or partial servings you can have and still stay within your diet guidelines for that meal.

3. It helps you compare food items and decide which are the best for your diet plan.

As you shop, compare items to find the best ones for your needs. Keep these facts in mind:

- "No sugar added" doesn't mean a product is sugar-free.
- "Fat free" means that the product contains less than 1/2 gram of fat per serving.
- "Low fat" means the product contains 3 grams of fat or less per serving.
- "Reduced fat" or "less fat" means 25 percent less fat than the regular version.

Keep in mind that foods promoted as being lower in fat may still contain harmful saturated fats and trans fats, and that the calories per serving are often about the same as in the regular version. Read the nutrition label to find out how much fat, what kind of fat, and how many calories the food contains. Low-carbohydrate foods are becoming popular, but they may contain more fat and the same amount or more calories as the regular version.

Begin with Small Changes

Don't try to change all of your eating habits at once. Here are some ways you can begin:

- Try fat-free or low-fat cheese, milk, and yogurt. Also try leaner cuts of meat. This will help you cut down on saturated fat without changing all of your food choices right away.
- Work measured portions of brown rice, other whole grains, and whole-wheat pasta into more meals. However, these foods will still raise your blood glucose. Testing your glucose level after eating these foods is the best way to tell if you should continue eating them.

• Eat more fresh vegetables. Frozen vegetables are better than canned.

• Avoid processed foods as much as possible; they tend to be high in trans fats, sugar, and sodium and low in fiber.

• Try tofu, soy milk, or vegetarian alternatives to meat products. (Substitutes such as these can help you cut cholesterol and saturated fat from your diet.)

Eating Out

Those with diabetes need not sacrifice the pleasure of going out to eat. Knowing about the different food groups and which foods to avoid or limit will help you make the right choices when you dine out; paying attention to serving sizes will keep you from eating too much. Here are some tips to help you choose the best foods:

• Before you order something, ask the server how it is prepared. Is it fried, baked, or grilled? If the normal method isn't a healthy choice for you, can it be cooked another way? Is it served in a heavy sauce—and, if so, can the chef omit the sauce or serve it on the side?

• Choose fish, lean meat, or skinless chicken that is broiled, poached, baked, or grilled.

• Order salads and steamed vegetables to accompany your meal. Request low-fat dressings and sauces; to control the amount of these you receive, ask to have them served on the side.

• Ask the server to suggest low-fat dishes. Restaurants nowadays encounter people on special diets all the time and will usually accommodate their customers.

• If you take insulin and know that your meal will be delayed, be sure to time your injection accordingly. You can eat a roll or a piece of fruit to tide you over and prevent hypoglycemia.

• If everyone around you is ordering dessert and you crave it, ask to share with someone. Even a few bites of a dessert can satisfy your urge.

Shun Super-Sizing

Restaurant portions are often much larger than what most of us need to eat or should eat. When the portions are huge, it's tempting to eat more than the amount that's right for you. Here are some tips to help you avoid eating too much:

- Ask your server about the size of an item. Is it big enough for two? Can you get a half order?
- Before you order, ask to see what a small, medium, or large size looks like.
- Choose smaller portions if they are offered—or order from the appetizer menu, where servings are usually smaller.
- Order half a sandwich and half a salad.
- Avoid buffets and "all you can eat" dishes.
- If you are served more than your meal plan allows, take the rest home for another time. If you tend to clean your plate, ask for a take-home box at the beginning of the meal and put the excess food in the box before you start eating.
- Ask the waiter not to serve bread.

Tips for Eating Out in Various Restaurants

The following list includes selections of healthy food choices from various cuisines. Remember to count the carbohydrates in each and eat only the amount that fits into your meal plan—half or less of a hamburger bun, one instead of two slices of bread for a sandwich, or just a few bites of a high-carbohydrate dish. Remember, you don't have to clean your plate. If you fear your willpower might waiver, ask the waiter to bring you half a serving—or omit an item altogether.

Asian

- Stir-fried fish, chicken, or lean beef with vegetables
- Sashimi (Japanese raw fish). Mix your own sauce of soy sauce and wasabi and leave out sweet ginger.
- "Hot pots" and other soups that contain lean meat, tofu, and vegetables. Hold the rice or ask for a small serving on the side.

Mexican
- Chicken or fish fajitas, but limit the beans, rice, and tortillas.
- Baked or broiled fish, seafood, or chicken dishes

Steak house (many now serve grilled fish as well)
- Grilled or broiled lean cuts of beef (round steak, sirloin, filet mignon, London broil, tip roast)
- Broiled or baked chicken breast (don't eat the skin)
- Steamed vegetables

Salad bars and buffets
- Lettuce; plain, fresh vegetables; beans with light dressing
- Roast chicken or turkey breast (without the skin) or sliced lean roast beef
- Steamed vegetables
- Fresh fruit (but pay attention to their carbohydrate content)

Fast food
Believe it or not, most fast-food restaurants will provide nutrition information if you ask. You can also check the Internet or various printed sources. Once again, watch the carbohydrates. Good choices include:
- Garden salad with light dressing
- Broiled, roasted, or grilled chicken sandwich; eat only half of the bun.
- Sliced turkey or lean roast beef sandwich without mayonnaise; make it an open-face sandwich, and eat only part of the bread.
- Grilled hamburger with bun, tomato, lettuce, pickles, onion, ketchup, and mustard (no cheese or "secret sauce"; eat only part of the bun)
- Avoid beverages high in sugar or fats, such as milkshakes.

What About Sugar and Alcohol?

Alcohol and sugar were once considered dangerous for people with diabetes, but it has since been established that small amounts will not necessarily interfere with wise diabetes management. Most people with either type of diabetes can eat some sugar, so long as they count it as a carbohydrate. (Always count the calories and monitor the carbohydrates in your daily meal plan.) You also can drink alcohol in moderation, as defined below. Although alcohol does not increase blood sugar, many alcoholic drinks happen to contain large amounts of sugar. For example, bourbon contains a lot of sugar, vodka almost none, and most mixed drinks have a great deal of sugar, largely from the mixers. White wine has a little sugar. Red wine has very little. Beer contains large amounts of carbohydrates, which will increase blood sugar.

Moderate amounts of alcohol can lower your risk of heart disease, but you need to be aware of what "moderate" means. For men, it equals two standard drinks a day; for women, one. A standard drink is:

- Beer: 12 ounces
- Wine: 5 ounces
- 80-proof distilled liquor: 1.5 ounces

Some of the effects of alcohol, such as drowsiness or slurred speech, resemble the symptoms of hypoglycemia (see box, page 43.) This means you could be experiencing hypoglycemia but mistake the symptoms for tipsiness from the alcohol. Also, if you are intoxicated, you may not notice the symptoms of low or high blood sugar. In some people, alcohol, especially on an empty stomach, can cause a low-glucose reaction.

Eat to Stay Healthy

If you have diabetes, it's up to you to manage your diet just as you manage other aspects of your health. By learning to choose the right foods—and by learning to balance them with your blood-glucose levels—you can enjoy meals and maintain a healthy lifestyle.

Work closely with your health care team as you develop your meal plan and learn to eat well. Your doctor and dietitian can teach you how to choose foods, how to eat balanced meals and snacks, and how to avoid swings in your blood-glucose levels that could usher in hypoglycemia or hyperglycemia.

8

Exercise and Physical Activity

E xercise is vital to good health. Exercise helps control weight, lower blood pressure, decrease bad cholesterol, and raise good cholesterol. It strengthens muscles and bones, improves circulation, reduces stress, and keeps your joints flexible.

For people with diabetes, physical activity is especially beneficial. It lowers blood-glucose levels and increases the body's sensitivity to insulin. This is a crucial advantage in type 2 diabetes, where insulin resistance is a problem, but people with type 1 diabetes benefit greatly from exercise too. A regular exercise program may help some people with type 2 diabetes lose weight and decrease—or even phase out—insulin or oral medication use. Exercise can also help prevent or delay the onset of type 2 diabetes, particularly in people at high risk for the disease, and it can reduce the risk of diabetic complications. Exercise also stimulates circulation and helps keep the heart strong.

Here are some ways exercise improves your health:

- Mental health: Physical activity relieves stress and helps you sleep better. It can also give you a greater sense of well-being.
- Blood glucose: Exercising drives glucose into muscle cells, helping you improve your blood-glucose levels. This may free you to use less medication to manage your diabetes.
- Weight: You can lose fat, gain muscle, and maintain a healthy weight by being more active. Less fat usually means better glucose control.
- Heart health: Being active can reduce your risk of heart disease and high blood pressure. It can also improve your cholesterol levels.

• Small blood vessels: Exercise can lower blood glucose (high blood glucose damages the walls of small blood vessels, which can cause eye, kidney, or nerve problems). Exercise also stimulates good circulation, helping to keep your small arteries and capillaries clear.

• Large blood vessels: Physical activity can improve the health of large blood vessels. This may mean better blood flow and fewer foot and leg problems.

Exercise and Blood Glucose

When you exercise, your body consumes glucose and other nutrients. As muscles exhaust their store of carbohydrates, the body takes glucose from the blood. This process goes on after you've stopped exercising because your muscles continue to remove glucose from the blood to restock their own supplies.

If you take insulin or certain types of diabetes pills, there are several ways in which increased physical activity can cause hypoglycemia— a condition in which your blood-glucose levels fall to abnormally low levels, risking a hypoglycemic reaction. (For a full list of the symptoms of hypoglycemia, see the box on page 43. Additionally, chapter 10 presents a detailed explanation of hypoglycemia and the urgency of treating it promptly.) If you have just taken an insulin injection or diabetes pills, the muscles you are exercising will take in more glucose than usual. Thus, your blood sugar will fall. If the level falls too much, you will develop hypoglycemia. Also, if you inject insulin into a muscle that's being used in the exercise, that muscle can absorb the insulin faster than when you're not exercising, thereby getting the insulin into your blood more quickly than you expected.

None of this means you shouldn't exercise; it simply means you must check your blood-glucose levels and adjust your carbohydrate intake accordingly. If you find that you are getting hypoglycemic when exercising, you may need to modify how much insulin or oral medication you take or the time at which you take it. If you go running, avoid taking your insulin in the buttocks or thighs. If you are lifting weights, avoid taking it in your arm.

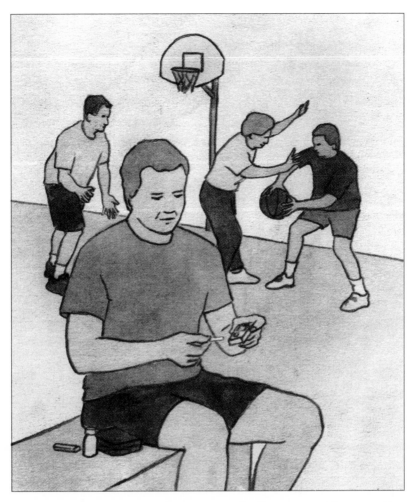

> Check blood sugar before and after exercise as directed by your health care provider.

First Stop on the Road to Fitness

Before you begin an exercise program or ratchet up an existing physical activity, check your plans with your health care provider. This is true for everyone—not just people with diabetes. It is especially vital if you are overweight, if you have a history of heart disease, or if you have diabetic neuropathy or peripheral vascular disease. Your health care provider may ask you to take a stress test to see how your heart responds to activity.

Exercise Safely

Physical activity must be safe in order for you to embrace it as a lifestyle. Generally, it is best to exercise one to three hours after eating, because that's when your blood-glucose levels tend to be higher. If you take insulin, sulfonylureas, or meglinitides, check your blood glucose before you exercise. If it is below 120 mg/dL, have a carbohydrate serving (such as a piece of fruit or a small snack) to boost the glucose level and stave off hypoglycemia. Test again 30 minutes later to see if your glucose levels are stable—that is, if they are pretty much the same, or if they have changed a lot.

You should likewise check your blood glucose after any vigorous exercise. Why? Because for people who take insulin and certain diabetes pills, the risk of hypoglycemia is often highest several hours after exercising.

People with diabetes should always wear a medical alert bracelet. If you take insulin or diabetes pills, the bracelet should say so. Also carry hard candy or glucose tablets with you when you exercise; should you begin to experience the symptoms of hypoglycemia, you can pop a few of these in your mouth to fight it off.

The Best Workout Plan for You

One key to becoming fit is to pace yourself. Start with activities you know you can handle at a level of exertion and for a duration that you can tolerate. Then, add other activities, gradually increasing your pace and duration. You may start by simply moving around a bit more. As your comfort level rises, you can increase your physical activity. You don't have to drive yourself to the brink of exhaustion to benefit from exercise. Here are some tips to keep in mind:

- Try to exercise for at least 20 to 30 minutes a day, five or more days a week. You may not be able to accomplish this at first, but you can always work your way up in duration and intensity.
- Include exercises that improve strength and flexibility, such as gentle stretching, as well as aerobic exercise (exercise that increases your heart rate and breathing).

• The saying "No pain, no gain" is nonsense. The best fitness plan is the one that matches your abilities.

Once you've added some activity to your day, you can become even more active. Remember, the key to maintaining an exercise plan is choosing something you like to do.

Make Your Activity Fun

Making exercise fun can help you stick to your plan. You needn't pick a strenuous exercise, nor do you have to join a gym or a health club. Simply find something you enjoy doing. You may like to walk, play tennis, dance, bike, or swim—or some combination of these. Try to exercise at least 20 to 30 minutes a day, five or more days per week.

Try these tips to make each workout welcome:

• Choose activities you enjoy doing.
• Involve your family or friends in your physical activity.
• Join a social club that goes for walks or does other physical activities.
• Try something new for you, for example, kayaking, rowing, or hiking.
• Dance! Jitterbug and Cajun dancing can be quite a workout. Even waltzing can provide aerobic exercise.

Keep It Simple

You don't have to make physical activity hard on yourself. Instead, find activities that fit easily into your schedule. Besides getting 20 to 30 minutes of exercise five or more days a week, increasing the amount of exercise you get from everyday activities can greatly improve your health. Here are some simple ways to add exercise to your day:

• Run small shopping errands on your bike, or walk to the grocery store.
• Get off the bus a stop or two early and walk the rest of the way.
• When you reach the parking lot of your destination, park your car in the space farthest from the door.

- Go for a 10-minute walk after each meal.
- Take the stairs instead of the elevator when you can.
- Go for a walk around the mall or shopping center before you begin shopping.

Build Up to Brisk Exercise

Whereas it is true that very sedentary people will benefit from doing just a little more, a real benefit for all people—especially diabetics— comes from exercise that modestly increases heart rate and is sustained for at least 20 minutes. So once you become more active, you may want to increase the pace. Again, choose an exercise you enjoy. Then check with your health care provider to be sure the exercise you have in mind will be safe for you.

The Benefits of Briskness

Brisk activity gets your heart beating faster. If you are walking or jog- ging, for example, imagine you are hurrying to an appointment—then

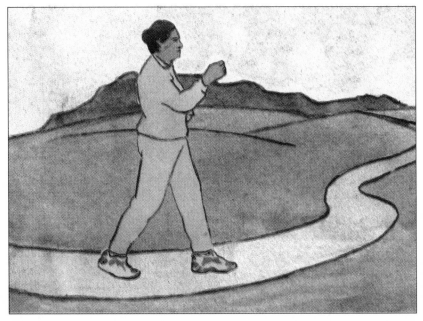

> Walking briskly (4 mph) for an hour can burn more than 400 calories.

walk or run commensurately faster. This can help you increase your fitness, lose extra weight, and manage your blood-glucose levels. If you have foot or leg problems, take up swimming, water aerobics at the local Y, or cycling. No matter what your activity, work up to 20 to 30 minutes of steady, brisk exercise on five or more days each week.

Warm Up and Cool Down

Warm up before you exercise and cool down afterward. This means doing a mild version of your activity for five or 10 minutes before and after your exercise routine. For example, when you set out for a walk, go slowly for the first 10 minutes or so, and then accelerate to a brisk pace. Warming up will gradually raise your body temperature and get your muscles, tendons, ligaments, and cardiovascular system ready for the movement that your exercise will entail. Cooling down does the reverse, gradually reducing your muscle temperature, which can prevent stiffness and soreness.

Stretch

Stretching is great for your body. It improves your flexibility, the range of motion of your joints, and your posture, and it helps relieve stress. It also can prevent injury to the muscles you use in your exercise. It's easier to injure or pull a muscle if it's cold, so it is often better to stretch after you finish exercising when your muscles are warm. If you do stretch before exercising, be sure to warm up first.

Take the Talk-Sing Test

The talk-sing test is a simple way to tell how hard you're exercising. If you can talk while exercising, you're in a safe range. But if you're out of breath and can't talk, slow down. If you can carry a tune, on the other hand, it's time to pick up the pace: Walk up a hill rather than on flat ground, increase the resistance on your stationary bike, or swim faster.

When to Halt an Activity

Stop exercising and call your health care provider right away if you notice any of the following:

- Pain, pressure, tightness, or heaviness in the chest
- Pain or heaviness in the neck, shoulders, back, arms, legs, or feet
- Unusual shortness of breath
- Dizziness or light-headedness
- Unusually rapid or slow pulse
- Increased joint or muscle pain
- Symptoms of hypoglycemia.

If these recur, talk to your doctor or nurse educator about adjusting your medicines.

Caring for Active Feet

Because you have diabetes, your feet require special care. Ask your health care provider to examine your feet to be sure it's okay to start being more active. Even if your doctor gives you the go-ahead to start exercising, check your feet daily to ensure there are no problems, such

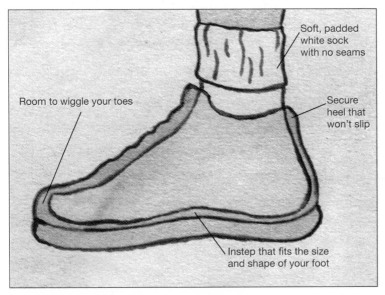

Soft, padded white sock with no seams

Room to wiggle your toes

Secure heel that won't slip

Instep that fits the size and shape of your foot

> Choose a shoe that fits correctly to avoid injuries.

as cuts, sores, blisters, red areas, rashes, or ingrown toenails, that exercise will aggravate (we discuss foot care in chapter 11.)

Properly fitted footwear is essential for anyone who exercises regularly. But it's even more important for people with diabetes, who are more likely to have nerve damage that can affect their feet. This nerve damage can cause peripheral neuropathy, a condition that may make your feet less sensitive to irritation and pain. If your shoes don't fit correctly, you could develop blisters or other foot problems but be unable to feel them right away. Poor circulation makes healing harder for people with diabetes, so recovering from even the simplest foot injury—a blister, for example—can be difficult.

Footwear basics

Proper footwear helps keep your feet healthy. Follow these guidelines:

- Wear the proper shoe for your activity. A running shoe, for instance, is specifically designed to keep your feet injury-free while jogging.
- Choose a shoe that gives your toes room to wiggle but does not let your heel slip. Your foot should also fit comfortably within the instep.
- Wear soft, seamless, well-padded socks.
- Dry your feet before putting on your socks and shoes.
- Get rid of your old, worn-out shoes. If the soles are thin and the shoes have lost their bounce, it's time to go shoe-shopping.
- As mentioned above, check your feet before and after your activity for cuts, sores, blisters, red areas, rashes, or ingrown toenails.

If You Have Diabetes-Related Eye Problems

If you have severe diabetic eye disease, be sure to ask your doctor which kinds of exercise are safe for your eyes. Your health care provider may advise you not to participate in certain exercises, such as jogging, diving, boxing, or weight lifting. These may cause the blood vessels in your eyes to bleed.

Fill in a Fitness Log

Record the information that matters most to you in a fitness log. This may document how you feel before, during, or after exercise. You can also jot down your blood-glucose levels. As time goes on, compare your first entry with more recent ones: Are your blood-glucose levels coming down? Is your overall feeling of fitness going up?

Date	Minutes	Blood-glucose level / Comments
5/18	25	

> Here is a sample of a fitness log that you can keep in a notebook or on a calendar. Record your walks and blood-glucose levels every day. This helps track your progress. Even noting that you didn't walk and why helps you notice patterns.

Safety Tips

Here are some general tips for exercising safely if you have diabetes:

- Check your blood sugar often.
- Carry identification.
- Wear a medical alert bracelet that says you have diabetes. (If you take insulin, the bracelet should note this as well.)
- Exercise with a friend so you're not alone.
- Use the proper footwear and safety equipment for your activity.
- Dress appropriately for the weather.
- Drink water before, during, and after exercise.
- Don't exercise in very hot or very cold weather.
- Don't exercise if you are sick.
- Carry a source of sugar to treat low blood sugar.
- Be sure to warm up before exercising and cool down afterward.
- Stretch to prevent muscle injury.
- Stop if you experience any of the symptoms listed at the top of page 106.

9

Complementary and Alternative Medicine

I f you are thinking of trying complementary or alternative medicine (CAM) for your diabetes, you are not alone. According to some studies, Americans make more trips to CAM practitioners than they do to their primary care physicians. They also spend more money on CAM remedies than they do for conventional medical care.

In addition, there happens to be greater interest in CAM among people with diabetes than there is among the general population: Some surveys have shown that people with diabetes (particularly those over 65) are more than twice as likely to use CAM treatments as are those without the disease. Simply because a lot of people are interested in such treatments, however, does not validate their efficacy.

Complementary? Alternative? Know the Difference

"Complementary medicine" and "alternative medicine" are broad terms used to describe a variety of treatments that fall outside the realm of traditional Western medicine. Before considering the treatments themselves, it is crucial to understand the difference between complementary and alternative.

A **complementary treatment** is one used in addition to a standard medical treatment. You may practice biofeedback, for example, or take herbal supplements as well as taking the conventional medications your doctor prescribes. In this case, the biofeedback or the supplement is said to complement, or enhance, your standard medical treatment. Be aware, though, that any complementary treatment or supplement you partake of could possibly interfere with, rather than optimize, your

The majority of studies and clinical trials designed to assess the safety and viability of complementary and alternative treatments have looked at only very small numbers of test subjects. They therefore cannot be used to claim efficacy, lack of it, or safety—nor should you put credence in them if they do. Tellingly, there is currently no non-FDA-approved compound that can be recommended to treat any form of diabetes.

medical treatment. That's why you will find the following statement reinforced several times throughout this chapter: Before you try any complementary or alternative treatment, discuss it with your health care provider to be certain it will not negatively affect your diabetes—or your health overall.

An **alternative treatment** is one that a person uses instead of a traditional prescription medication or treatment. The danger here should be obvious: Diabetes medications and insulin are carefully designed to help your body balance its blood-glucose levels in order to maintain your good health. These medications are made available to the general public only after thorough scientific research and testing have demonstrated their safety and effectiveness. Replacing your diabetes medication or insulin with an alternative treatment that has not undergone this rigorous testing could thus potentially have devastating results for your health. Talk to your health care provider before trying *any* alternative treatment.

Because of the American public's growing interest in CAM, the National Institutes of Health established a special division, the National Center for Complementary and Alternative Medicine (NCCAM), to study the safety and efficacy of these treatments. Another part of the NCCAM mandate is to furnish the most current information available on complementary and alternative medicine. NCCAM's website (http://nccam.nih.gov/) serves as an excellent resource for anyone seeking to explore CAM treatments.

Research-based knowledge about CAM is steadily growing. Many CAM therapies—notably some herbal and mineral supplements—are undergoing clinical trials to determine their value. Although some evidence suggests that certain complementary treatments may benefit people with diabetes, discuss them in advance with your health care pro-vider to make certain they won't harm you.

Commonly Used Uncommon Treatments

Many different types of therapy may be considered complementary or alternative, and any list of these therapies would likely go on for pages. Merely identifying those that are most frequently sought out by people with diabetes would be difficult if not impossible. Many CAM treatments—massage and biofeedback, to cite two stalwarts—are designed to treat any illness, not just focus on a single ailment. Indeed, certain CAM treatments pursued by people with diabetes are based on the idea of treating the entire body—the whole person—rather than one illness. Here are a few you may encounter in your reading.

Acupuncture is a traditional Chinese medicine based on the concept of a vital energy that flows throughout the body. A practitioner inserts needles into designated points on the skin to heal certain ailments. Some scientists believe that acupuncture triggers the release of the body's natural painkillers; it has been shown to offer relief from some forms of pain. People with neuropathy—the painful nerve disease of diabetes—sometimes use acupuncture.

Biofeedback is an alternative therapy that emphasizes relaxation and stress-reduction techniques, helping a person become more aware of—and learn to deal with—the body's response to pain. It has proved effective in treating high blood pressure, stress and anxiety, insomnia, and overeating. Beyond its demonstrated ability to help people curb their appetites, however, not a shred of evidence exists to indicate that biofeedback is useful as a diabetes treatment.

Dietary supplements can include vitamins, minerals, herbs, and animal products. They come in many forms—including tablets, powders, or liquids—and are sold in grocery stores, health food stores, and pharmacies. Dietary supplements are often marketed as "natural" remedies. Merely because something is natural, however, does not mean it is effective—or even safe. Because supplements are regulated as food and not as drugs according to the FDA's definition of the term, that agency has only limited power to regulate them. Dietary supplements can interact with prescribed and over-the-counter drugs, as well as with other supplements.

Guided imagery is a relaxation technique employed by some professionals who also use biofeedback. With guided imagery, a person thinks of peaceful mental images, such as ocean waves. As part of this exercise, the person may also visualize scenes of controlling or curing a chronic disease, such as diabetes. People using this technique believe the positive images can ease their condition.

Mind-body medicine uses a variety of techniques to enhance the mind's capacity to affect bodily function and symptoms. These techniques include meditation, prayer, mental healing, and therapies involving art, music, or dance. Some mind-body techniques that were considered CAM in the past—patient-support groups, for example—have since moved into the mainstream.

Naturopathy is a field of alternative medicine in which practitioners claim to work with natural healing forces within the body, with the goal of helping the body heal itself from disease. Naturopathy's focus is on the whole person rather than on an isolated disease, such as diabetes. Practices may include dietary modifications, massage, acupuncture, and lifestyle changes.

Before You Take the Plunge

Always talk to your health care provider before trying any treatment or taking any supplements that he or she has not prescribed. In particular, do not stop your regular treatment and replace it with an alternative therapy; this could risk your health and well-being. Because many people anticipate that their health care providers will not approve of CAM, they hesitate to bring it up with them. In reality, most doctors are familiar with CAM therapies—or can easily find out about them. Your health care provider can advise you about which ones are safe and which ones might interfere with your treatment, thus causing health problems.

But Do They Work?

Most of the available information about complementary and alternative therapies comes from patients who report that a certain treatment worked for them. Often there is no scientific evidence to support these claims. Although some studies are under way to evaluate the safety and effectiveness of various CAM therapies, the results have been conflicting so far. When one study shows that a certain CAM therapy is effective, another study is just as likely to show that it is not.

So... how can you tell that a given CAM treatment is worth investigating? You should talk to your health care provider before trying any new treatment, of course, but you may also want to do some research on your own to discover more about the therapy in question. One critical question to answer as you read and learn is this: Has a treatment been scientifically evaluated in a clinical study?

Clinical Studies

Clinical studies, also called clinical trials, are research studies conducted among human volunteers to evaluate the effectiveness of new methods of preventing or treating diseases. Every new prescription drug that appears in U.S. pharmacies must, by law, undergo clinical studies to determine that it is both safe and effective for humans.

In considering a CAM treatment, one of the first steps is to find out if the treatment you are investigating has been studied in humans with your medical condition. There are two types of clinical trials:

1. Interventional trials investigate whether a new treatment (or a new way of using a known treatment) is safe and effective.
2. Observational trials examine health issues besetting large groups of people or populations.

The results of clinical trials are usually reported in peer-reviewed medical journals. If a study appears in a peer-reviewed journal, it means its validity has been assessed by an independent panel of medical experts (peers). Examples of such journals include the *New England Journal of Medicine* and the *Journal of the American Medical Association*.

You can search through peer-reviewed literature in a medical library or at www.pubmed.gov. At this website, you simply type in the name of the treatment you want to learn about; the database then presents a list of relevant articles, along with a summary of the articles, if available.

What About Dietary Supplements?

Although researchers are studying some dietary supplements to see if they can help people with diabetes control their blood-glucose levels, no conclusive evidence is available at this time to recommend or exclude any supplement. Below you will find a summary of several dietary supplements that claim to be beneficial in the treatment of diabetes.

Alpha-Lipoic Acid

Alpha-lipoic acid (ALA) is an antioxidant—a supplement similar to a vitamin—that prevents cell damage. Some evidence indicates that ALA may be of use in lowering blood-glucose levels. Foods such as liver, broccoli, spinach, and potatoes all contain ALA. The substance is also sold as tablets or capsules.

In 2003, the Mayo Clinic conducted a study of ALA with a medical center in Russia. The study suggested that ALA can reduce the frequency and severity of the most common symptoms of diabetic neuropathy, including burning and sharp pain, prickling sensations, and numbness. However, the ALA used in the study was administered by intravenous injection. The results may not be the same with tablets, the only form available for sale at this time.

Researchers continue to study this supplement to learn more about how it can possibly combat diabetes.

Chromium

Chromium is a metal and a trace mineral that the body requires to make glucose-tolerance factor—a dietary compound that has been linked to maintaining glucose tolerance. Many foods contain chromium, including meats, fish, coffee, tea, some whole-grain breads, and brewer's yeast.

It is also sold as capsules and tablets labeled chromium picolinate, chromium chloride, or chromium nicotinate.

Some studies have shown that chromium has no beneficial effects for people with diabetes. Others suggest that it lowers blood-glucose levels. Although researchers continue to study its safety and effectiveness, not enough evidence is available at this time to recommend chromium for the treatment of diabetes.

Taking chromium in low doses for a short period of time appears to be safe for most adults. Side effects are weight gain, headache, sleep problems, skin irritation, and worsening of mood disorders. A major concern in diabetes is that chromium may cause kidney problems.

Cinnamon

Some studies from a few years ago found that ground cinnamon appeared to have a beneficial effect on blood glucose and that it lowered cholesterol and triglyceride levels. In these studies, cinnamon seemed to stimulate the production of glucose-burning enzymes, which increase insulin's effectiveness in regulating blood sugar. Subsequent studies, however, have called into question whether cinnamon has any beneficial effect on blood-glucose levels.

Coenzyme Q10

Coenzyme Q10, also called CoQ10, ubiquinone, or ubiquinol, is similar to a vitamin. It helps cells make energy and acts as an antioxidant—a substance that prevents cell damage. Meat and seafood contain CoQ10. It is also sold in tablets and capsules. There is no evidence that CoQ10 has any effect in controlling blood glucose. (Theoretically, it may have some benefit against heart disease, but more research is needed to determine if this is so.) CoQ10 appears to be safe in general, although it may interact with other medicines, including some blood thinners.

Fenugreek

Fenugreek is an aromatic plant native to Asia and southern Europe. Its seeds are used whole or ground to flavor foods, such as Indian curries, teas, and spice mixtures. In many Middle Eastern countries, it is used to make tea. It is also sold as an herbal supplement.

In clinical studies, fenugreek displayed anti-diabetic properties: It improved glucose tolerance in both type 2 and type 1 diabetes. Scientists continue to explore its potential in treating diabetes.

Ginseng

Several types of plants are referred to as ginseng, but most studies of ginseng and diabetes have looked at American ginseng. These studies have shown that ginseng marginally lowers both fasting and after-meal blood-glucose levels. American ginseng also has been shown to lower three-month average blood-glucose levels, or HbA1c.

Magnesium

Magnesium is a mineral found in leafy green vegetables, nuts, seeds, and some whole grains. It is also sold as tablets, capsules, and liquids. Magnesium is vital to the smooth functioning of several key body systems, including heart, nerves, muscles, and bones. People with diabetes commonly have low levels of magnesium.

Despite the existence of a few studies on magnesium and diabetes, researchers do not yet fully understand the relationship between the mineral and the disease. For starters, they know that a magnesium deficiency may increase insulin resistance. They also know that low magnesium may impair insulin secretion by the pancreas, which can foster certain diabetic complications.

Low doses of magnesium supplements appear to be safe for most people—except those with kidney problems. In high doses, however, magnesium may cause nausea, diarrhea, appetite loss, low blood pressure, irregular heart rate, muscle weakness, and confusion. The mineral can also interact unfavorably with other drugs.

Talk to Your Doctor

Whether you have diabetes or another disease, it is critical that you talk to your doctor, educator, or other health care provider before you try any complementary or alternative therapy. Remember, a complementary treatment should enhance your regular medical care, not replace it, and its benefits should outweigh its risks. Many CAM treatments contain ingredients that can interfere with your regular therapy, making your physical condition worse.

Be very specific, therefore, when you discuss with your doctor any CAM treatment you may be contemplating. Ask her or him about its potential dangers or advantages. You'll also have to weigh the cost of complementary treatment and determine whether your health insurance plan will cover the one you are considering. Health insurance coverage for CAM is often limited; not only that, but it varies according to your state of residence.

It's never a bad idea to educate yourself before you talk to your doctor. You can research a CAM therapy you're interested in, either in a library or on a reputable website such as these four sponsored by the National Institutes of Health:

nccam.nih.gov/health/decisions
nccam.nih.gov/health/diabetes
http://nccam.nih.gov/health/financial/
diabetes.niddk.nih.gov/dm/pubs/alternativetherapies/

As with every other aspect of diabetes care, you are in charge of your treatment, so it makes sense to be an "educated commander." The optimal way to manage your diabetes is to make informed treatment decisions in close consultation with your health care providers.

10

Hypoglycemia

anaging diabetes is a delicate balancing act—keeping your blood-glucose levels as near normal as possible while simultaneously fending off hypoglycemia, a condition in which those levels fall dangerously low.

Whether you have been diagnosed with diabetes recently or have lived with the ailment for years, hypoglycemia—the subject of this chapter—can develop with surprising ease. It can occur if you take too much medication, delay or skip a meal, or exercise more vigorously or longer than usual. Even when you closely monitor your diet, exercise, medication, and blood glucose, your glucose levels can occasionally slip out of balance. This chapter explains how to prepare for this possibility so you will know how to handle it when it happens.

Hypoglycemia is less common with type 2 diabetes than with type 1, but it can be a problem with both. Know the signs of hypoglycemia, and take action to treat it right away.

Symptoms of Hypoglycemia

In general, hypoglycemia can happen when your blood-sugar levels fall below 60 mg/dL or drop rapidly from high to low. Some people experience no symptoms until their levels are below 60 mg/dL, however. Some have symptoms when their levels are higher.

When blood glucose drops too low, the body tries to protect itself by activating several "rescue" mechanisms. The most important is the release of adrenaline from the adrenal glands, which raises blood glucose. This adrenaline surge makes you feel anxious, sweaty, and lightheaded. In addition, your heart beats more rapidly and forcefully, which you may sense as palpitations. You may also feel hungry or nauseated. Because of these symptoms, most people awaken from sleep if they develop hypoglycemia; if they don't, the reaction can be particularly dangerous. Such is sometimes the case when people have taken sleeping pills or have consumed a large amount of alcohol.

If blood glucose falls even lower, brain function can be affected. (In much the same way that a car runs on gasoline, the brain uses glucose as its fuel.) Deprived of glucose for too long, your brain may cause you to experience fatigue, weakness, blurred vision, and confusion. Blood-glucose levels that drop even further can induce loss of consciousness or seizures. Rarely—and sometimes with tragic consequences—people having a hypoglycemic reaction may be mistakenly viewed as drunk or on illegal drugs, with the result that they are blocked from receiving appropriate treatment.

Symptoms of hypoglycemia vary from person to person, but may include any of the following:

- Nervousness and shakiness
- Anxiety
- Difficulty concentrating
- Perspiration
- Pale skin
- Dizziness or light-headedness
- Palpitations
- Rapid heartbeat
- Shallow breathing
- Numbness of the mouth
- Tingling in the fingers
- Muscle weakness
- Tremors
- Blurred vision
- Sleepiness
- Confusion
- Difficulty speaking
- Hunger
- Loss of consciousness

If hypoglycemia comes on very quickly, as it occasionally does, you may lack the time to treat it before you become mentally confused or pass out. For this reason, it is crucial that you inform the people with whom you live and work that you have diabetes. Next, describe for them the symptoms of hypoglycemia. Finally, spell out precisely what they should do for you if they observe you exhibiting any of these symptoms.

People with diabetes should wear a medical alert bracelet. If you have a bout of hypoglycemia when you are with strangers, the bracelet will identify your condition and maximize your chances of receiving proper medical attention. If you take insulin or certain diabetes pills, the bracelet should specify their names.

What to Do

If you begin to feel symptoms of hypoglycemia, act quickly. You need to eat or drink some sugar that will enter your bloodstream quickly. The table on page 123 lists rapid-acting sources of sugar and the amount of sugar each one contains. In general, you want to consume 10 to 15 grams of quick sugar. Four to six ounces of fruit juice, half a can of regular (nondiet) soda, two tablespoons of raisins, or some candy will give you about that amount. (Surprisingly, perhaps, a glass of milk also works well.)

Most diabetics should carry fast-acting glucose tablets, which are sold in pharmacies. Each tablet usually contains about 4 grams of glucose, so you will need to chew and swallow three or four of them. Because the tablets contain glucose rather than sucrose (the more complex sugar found in most foods), they provide the fastest-acting sugar for treating hypoglycemia.

Here are some guidelines to follow for dealing with hypoglycemia:

• Check your blood sugar.
• Eat or drink 10 to 15 grams of fast-acting sugar (see table, page 123). Don't take more than this, or your blood sugar may climb too high. Typically, three or four glucose tablets will suffice; if none are available, consume half a cup (4 to 6 ounces) of fruit juice or nondiet soda, or 2 teaspoons of sugar or honey.

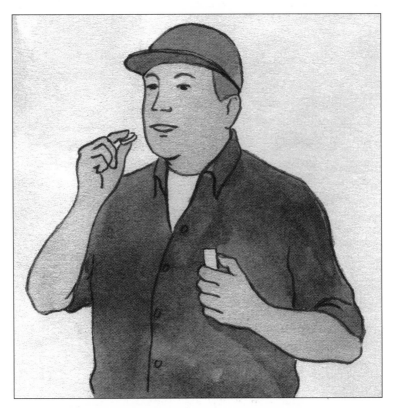

> If you take diabetes pills or insulin, always carry fast-acting sugar to treat low blood sugar.

• Wait 15 minutes, then recheck your blood sugar if you can. (If your symptoms are getting worse, don't wait the full 15 minutes before taking more sugar. You can always correct high blood sugar later.)

• If your blood sugar is still too low, repeat the steps above. If you aren't better after that, seek medical help.

• Remember that the increased level of adrenaline may cause symptoms of hypoglycemia even though your blood glucose has returned to a safe level. These symptoms may last another 10 or 15 minutes, but any confusion should dissipate right away.

• Once your blood sugar returns to the target range, have something to eat—but not just sugar. If your next meal is less than

When treating hypoglycemia, the following table will help you determine how much sugar to use.

Source of Sugar in Grams (g)	Amount to Use
Glucose tablets (1 tablet = 4-5g)	3-4 tablets
Glucose gel (31g tube)	½–⅔ tube
Cake icing (1 tsp = 4g)	4–5 teaspoons
Maple or corn syrup (1 tsp = 5g)	3–4 teaspoons
Orange or apple juice (⅓ cup = 10g)	½–1 cup
Table sugar (1 tsp = 4g)	4–5 teaspoons
Regular nondiet soda (⅙ cup = 3g)	¾ cup
Raisins (1 tbsp = 7½g)	2½–3 tablespoons
Life Savers (2 = 5g)	6–8 pieces
Milk: lowfat or skim (1 cup = 13g)	1 cup–1½ cups
Smarties (1 roll = 6-7g)	3 rolls
Sweet Tarts (each 1.7g)	8–12 pieces
Skittles (each 1g)	15–20 pieces

Use of trade names is for identification only and does not imply endorsement by AARP.

one hour away, eat that meal now. If it is more than an hour away, eat a snack—half a sandwich, perhaps, or some crackers and cheese.

• If you experience hypoglycemia several times, call your doctor.

If you have type 1 diabetes, your health care provider may recommend that you keep a glucagon-injection kit handy—perhaps one at home, one at work, and one in your car. (Keep in mind, however, that the interior of your vehicle tends to warm appreciably during the day, and that glucagon is not stable for long periods in heat.) An injection of glucagon—which is not a sugar but rather a chemical that causes your liver to rapidly release its stored carbohydrate—can help you recover from hypoglycemia by quickly boosting your blood-glucose levels.

In the event that your hypoglycemia is so severe you lose consciousness, you obviously won't be able to eat anything to treat it. Teach a family member or someone you work with how to give you the injection in this event.

Abrupt changes in diet, exercise, or medication can alter your blood-glucose levels as well. Before making any such adjustments, seek your physician's advice on how to keep your blood-glucose levels from dropping too low. And be aware that you may need to monitor your blood more often once you do make a change.

If you have diabetes and take insulin, you may need to check your blood-glucose levels in the middle of the night, usually at 3:00 a.m., to detect hypoglycemia. You may also have to check your levels before driving a car or engaging in other potentially dangerous activities. Your health care team can tell you how often to check.

Most people with type 2 or type 1 diabetes experience hypoglycemia at some time no matter how carefully they balance their diet, exercise, medication, and blood-glucose monitoring. If you have type 1 diabetes or frequent hypoglycemia, it is especially vital that you let the people around you know. That way, they can be prepared—and equipped—to come to your aid if they notice you showing the signs of this temporary but dangerous condition.

11

Long-Term Complications

People with diabetes can live normal, active lives if they practice good self-care and have the support of a high-quality health care team. If diabetes is not carefully managed, however, the resulting high blood-glucose levels can cause several serious health problems (described in this chapter), often without your knowing they are present until it is too late. For this reason, people with diabetes must pay careful attention to their blood-glucose level and control it carefully.

Precisely how high blood-sugar levels damage the body has yet to be puzzled out, but most researchers agree on the identity of at least one culprit: the accumulation of complex sugars within the walls of blood vessels. This buildup, scientists believe, changes the blood-vessel walls over time, ultimately making them thicken, lose their elasticity, and leak. As the walls get thicker, they clog the vessels' pathways, impeding blood flow to body organs. Deprived of their blood supply, vital organs cannot absorb all the nutrients and oxygen they need; as a result, they begin to function improperly.

Long-term problems—those that develop after a year or more of poorly controlled diabetes—include cardiovascular disease (including heart disease, stroke, and circulation problems), eye diseases, nerve damage, kidney disease, mouth infections, skin infections, and foot problems—occasionally so serious that they necessitate amputation. These health problems beset people with diabetes (both type 2 and type 1) more often than members of the general population.

Preventing Complications

From 1983 to 1993, the National Institutes of Health conducted a large scientific study called the Diabetes Control and Complications Trial (DCCT). The study's purpose: to learn if it is possible to prevent or reduce the health problems encountered by people with type 1 diabetes.

The DCCT brought good news: If people with type 1 diabetes carefully control their blood-glucose levels, they can reduce their risk of eye disease by 76 percent, nerve disease by 60 percent, and kidney disease by 50 percent. Scientists continue to analyze the DCCT results to learn more about how to prevent many of the health problems that accompany diabetes.

In 2005, the National Institutes of Health announced additional good news from the DCCT: People with type 1 diabetes who carefully control their blood-glucose levels can reduce their risk of heart disease and stroke by 50 percent. (Although the DCCT studied only people with type 1 diabetes, researchers believe that the findings apply to those with type 2 diabetes as well.)

Cardiovascular Disease

Among the most common (and the most severe) diabetic complications is cardiovascular disease. It can cause angina, heart attack, stroke, and leg pain from poor circulation and blocked arteries (conditions known collectively as peripheral artery disease). And poor circulation, in turn, can necessitate amputations.

As mentioned at the beginning of this chapter, people with diabetes are more prone to cardiovascular disease because diabetes thickens and damages blood vessels, which then become atherosclerotic, or clogged with plaque. Not only that, but people with diabetes—especially those with type 2—tend to have or develop other conditions or diseases that increase their risk for cardiovascular disease. These include high blood pressure, elevated "bad" cholesterol, high triglycerides, kidney disease, obesity, and susceptibility to blood clots. All of these afflictions boost a person's likelihood of developing cardiovascular disease.

If you have diabetes, you should understand the risk factors for cardiovascular disease. The main ones are these:

- High blood sugar
- High blood pressure (the blood pushes too hard against artery walls as it travels through the arteries)
- High levels of lipids (fatlike substances, such as cholesterol) in the blood
- Lack of exercise
- Smoking

Most people with diabetes have at least some of these risk factors. But, as the DCCT showed, you can reduce your risk of heart disease by controlling your blood-sugar levels. You can also make lifestyle changes to reduce your blood pressure and lipids. These changes include eating healthier foods, quitting smoking, and getting exercise. Medications may be needed as well.

Here's how these risk factors cause problems:

- High blood sugar. This situation causes the accretion of toxic substances in the walls of blood vessels. Once blood vessels become damaged, the interior artery walls become rough. Plaque then builds up—a condition known as atherosclerosis—constricting the flow of blood through the arteries. Having high blood sugar makes you more likely to have high blood pressure and high lipid levels.

- High blood pressure. When blood pressure is high, artery walls become damaged. Plaque is more likely to build up.

- High lipid levels. Lipids can include cholesterol, low-density lipoproteins (LDLs), and triglycerides—fats in the blood that the body needs to stay healthy. But lipid levels that are too elevated can damage the artery walls and allow plaque to form.

Certain other risk factors for heart disease stem from lifestyle decisions—or simply circumstances—that tend to raise your blood sugar, blood pressure, and lipids.

• Smoking. This activity damages the lining of your arteries, inviting plaque to build up on the artery walls. Smoking also narrows the arteries, which can raise blood pressure.

• Physical inactivity. Indolence keeps your heart from reaching its peak working condition. This can permit plaque to accumulate in the arteries. It also makes you more likely to have high blood pressure. Further, exercise stimulates blood flow through arteries; without exercise, you lose out on this preventive measure.

• Being overweight. Extra pounds make it harder for your body to use insulin. They make your heart work harder too.

Heart Disease

To understand why heart disease causes problems, it helps to know how your heart works. The heart is a muscle that pumps blood to the lungs, where the blood collects oxygen. The oxygen-rich blood then travels back to the heart and is pumped from there to the rest of the body. In order for the heart muscle to stay healthy, it must have a steady supply of oxygenated blood. This blood reaches the heart muscle through the coronary arteries.

The coronary arteries branch off from the aorta. (The body's main circulatory conduit, this large vessel delivers oxygen-rich blood from your heart to the rest of your body.) Branching off from the coronary arteries, in turn, are smaller arteries that thread their way over and through the heart muscle. These nourish every part of the heart with blood.

No matter where in the body they are located, healthy arteries have flexible walls and smooth inner linings. This allows blood to flow through them freely, carrying oxygen all over the body. The coronary arteries lie on the outside surface of the heart, so the blood flowing through them supplies oxygen to the heart muscle. The heart muscle needs this oxygen to stay healthy and to keep pumping blood throughout the body.

Heart disease is caused by atherosclerosis, or hardening of the arteries, which occurs when plaque (deposits of fat, cholesterol, and other

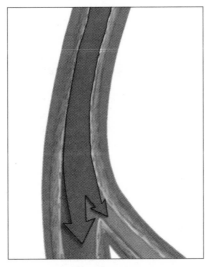

> **Healthy Artery.** The inner wall of a normal coronary artery is smooth. The artery is unblocked. Oxygen-rich blood flows easily to the heart muscle.

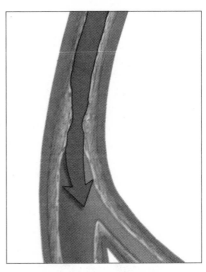

> **Damaged Artery.** High blood sugar, high blood pressure, and high levels of lipids damage artery walls. Plaque then collects on the damaged wall.

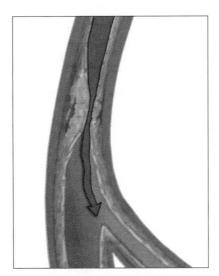

> **Narrowed Artery.** As more plaque builds up, the artery narrows. Blood flow to the heart is partly blocked. You may feel symptoms such as chest tightness or pain (angina).

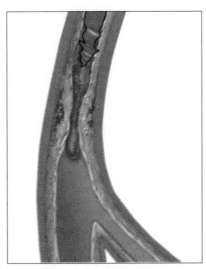

> **Blocked Artery.** When plaque or a blood clot (a mass of blood cells) fully blocks the artery, blood can't flow to the heart muscle. A heart attack may result.

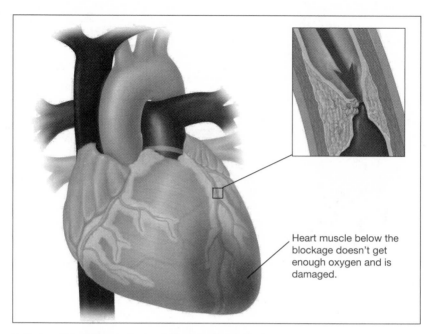

Heart muscle below the blockage doesn't get enough oxygen and is damaged.

> Reduced blood flow to the heart triggers a heart attack.

materials) collects along the arteries' inside walls. As plaque builds up, the arteries narrow; they can even become blocked. Blood flow is reduced, starving the heart of the oxygenated blood it must have to function smoothly. This deficit may trigger a heart attack—another name for damage to part of the heart muscle.

Sometimes plaque ruptures, or breaks open, spewing material downstream and potentially blocking the artery. When you have heart disease, these problems occur in the coronary arteries. That's why heart disease is also called coronary artery disease.

Arteries aren't vulnerable in the heart alone. Two other dangers are stroke (damage to an artery serving the brain) and peripheral artery disease (damage to an artery supplying the legs and feet). Taking steps to minimize your risk of heart disease can reduce your risk of arterial injury elsewhere in the body.

If you have heart disease, it's not too late to make a difference. By managing your risk factors and taking prescribed medications, you can avoid or postpone problems. Talk to your health care provider about reducing your risk of heart disease. If you've had a heart attack or other heart-related problem, make sure you understand why it happened—and what steps you can take now to stave off its recurrence.

Stroke

A stroke harms the brain the same way some heart attacks hurt the heart. During a stroke, blood cannot reach part of the brain. This may cause such symptoms as weakness in the face, arm, or leg, or trouble seeing or speaking. Seek medical attention immediately if you have any of these symptoms.

Diabetes is a risk factor for stroke, but other risk factors, when combined with diabetes, put you in even greater jeopardy. One of these is high blood pressure. Another is high cholesterol. Your lifestyle, too, can raise your risk—if you smoke, for example, if you drink more than two alcoholic beverages a day, or if you fail to exercise regularly. Overeating high-fat foods or being overweight or obese increases your risk as well.

Certain groups of people are at higher risk of stroke. Men are more prone to strokes than women. People over age 55 are at greater risk. And African Americans are more likely than whites to have a stroke.

You can lower your odds of having a stroke by quitting smoking, eating a healthy diet, exercising, and keeping your blood pressure and glucose within their normal range. Further, you should work with your health care team to control any health problems you may have and to learn the best ways of minimizing your risk.

Peripheral Artery Disease

Peripheral artery disease—also called peripheral vascular disease—is a type of cardiovascular disease in which your blood vessels become narrow or blocked and poor circulation prevents an adequate supply of blood from reaching your legs and feet. Peripheral artery disease is more common—and much more severe—in those with diabetes, but people without diabetes get it too. The disease is much worse in people who smoke. In people with diabetes, especially in those who smoke, the tiniest blood vessels, called capillaries, also are damaged. When capillary walls are abnormally thick, oxygen cannot get from the blood-

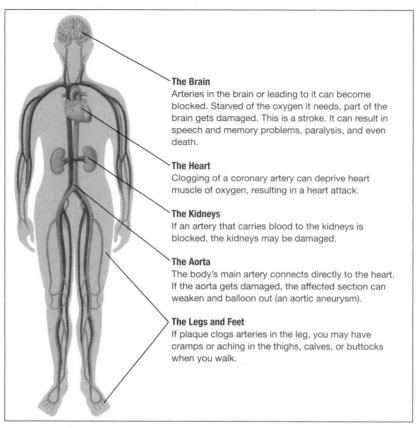

The Brain
Arteries in the brain or leading to it can become blocked. Starved of the oxygen it needs, part of the brain gets damaged. This is a stroke. It can result in speech and memory problems, paralysis, and even death.

The Heart
Clogging of a coronary artery can deprive heart muscle of oxygen, resulting in a heart attack.

The Kidneys
If an artery that carries blood to the kidneys is blocked, the kidneys may be damaged.

The Aorta
The body's main artery connects directly to the heart. If the aorta gets damaged, the affected section can weaken and balloon out (an aortic aneurysm).

The Legs and Feet
If plaque clogs arteries in the leg, you may have cramps or aching in the thighs, calves, or buttocks when you walk.

> Your whole body is at risk from plaque buildup.

stream to the tissues that need it. There's a double whammy: The bigger arteries don't supply enough blood, while the smallest arteries can't deliver the reduced amount of oxygen where it's needed. Some symptoms of peripheral artery disease include cramping or pain in the calves or thighs when walking. Occasionally leg pain can occur at night, which may be relieved by dangling the leg.

Peripheral artery disease blocks blood vessels large and small. For people with diabetes, the majority of problems usually stem from blockages in the arteries that supply blood to the thighs and legs. At first these blockages may cause no symptoms at all. As the disease progresses, however, you may experience a pain called claudication in your calves when you walk any distance or climb stairs. When the disease is advanced, the pain is noticeable even when a person is at rest, and the skin on the feet and lower legs may become black. If the skin becomes black, seek medical care immediately. Sometimes surgery becomes necessary to relieve the pain.

Because peripheral vascular disease impairs circulation to the legs and feet, injuries to those limbs heal slowly. Peripheral artery disease affects both legs, but one is usually affected more than the other.

Here are some of the measures you can take to prevent or control peripheral artery disease:

- Don't smoke. If you do smoke, quit.
- Keep your blood pressure under control.
- Keep your cholesterol and triglyceride levels normal.
- Keep your blood glucose as close to normal as possible.
- Exercise regularly.
- If you customarily consume more than two drinks per day, reduce your alcohol intake.

Peripheral artery disease can sometimes be treated with bypass surgery, in which a section of vein from another part of the body (or even an artificial vein) is transplanted to channel blood around the blocked artery and restore blood flow. This procedure is called a bypass. A blocked artery may also be opened by a less invasive procedure that uses a small balloon in a process called angioplasty. When these treatments fail or are not an option, amputation may be necessary.

Nerve Damage

Nerve damage, or neuropathy, affects people with diabetes in many ways. To understand the effects of nerve damage, it helps to understand how the nerves work.

Nerves operate in a network that sends signals to and from different parts of the body. When nerves are damaged, two things can happen: The signals may slow down or incorrect signals may be sent.

Scientists have figured out many of the mechanisms (if not all of the details) by which diabetes damages nerves. They are relatively certain, for example, that having high blood glucose causes a chemical imbalance in nerves or restricts blood flow to nerves.

Whatever its origin, the resulting nerve damage can cause several types of problems. It can change how your sensation works, causing numbness, tingling, a burning sensation, and a loss of sensitivity to touch. It can cause pain and problems with such basic functions as digestion and the workings of the bladder and bowel. Nerve damage also can interfere with sexual function and cause paralysis of a muscle.

People with diabetes can have three types of nerve damage: peripheral neuropathy, or nerve damage that affects the arms and legs; focal neuropathy, or nerve damage affecting a particular body part; and autonomic neuropathy, or damage to nerves that control involuntary body functions. All three types are explained in greater detail below.

Peripheral Neuropathy

Peripheral neuropathy is a type of nerve damage that affects the long nerves that run from your spine to your arms and legs. When these nerves are damaged, you experience numbness, tingling, and a loss of sensitivity to light touch. Sometimes you may even feel a burning, shooting, or stabbing pain.

Because this type of nerve damage makes you lose sensation to vibration, touch, and pain (especially in your feet), peripheral neuropathy can be dangerous. It means you could unwittingly injure your feet—from shoes that don't fit well, for instance, or from walking or some other form of exercise—and not realize it. If you also have poor circulation from peripheral artery disease, these injuries to your feet do

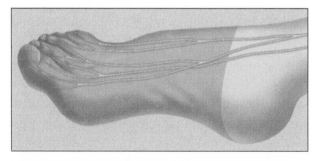

> Symptoms of neuropathy often begin in the toes and spread up the feet (shaded area).

not heal well and sores can become infected. If the infection is severe and cannot be healed, amputation may be necessary. For this reason, it is crucial for people with diabetes to pay close attention to their feet, checking regularly for injuries or sores they may be unable to feel. Expect your health care provider to check your feet at every visit—for sensation as well as for sores.

Focal Neuropathy

Focal neuropathy is damage to one nerve or a set of nerves. This damage can cause muscles to malfunction in the face, arms, legs, or eyes. If you have focal neuropathy, you may feel a weakness in your hand, have trouble lifting one of your legs, or experience double vision. The cause is probably blockages in a small blood vessel to the nerve, and the symptoms usually disappear after a few months. Carpal tunnel syndrome—a disorder of the nerves in the wrist—is perhaps the best-known example of focal neuropathy.

Autonomic Neuropathy

Autonomic neuropathy means damage to the autonomic nerves—those that control automatic body functions. Some examples of these critical processes include digestion, heartbeat, sweating, and sexual function. When autonomic nerves are damaged, a person can experience a range of unpleasant effects. Among these are profuse sweating, racing heartbeat, dizziness, nausea, vomiting, diarrhea, and sexual problems. The latter are discussed in detail in chapter 12.

Bladder Problems

Autonomic nerve damage can impair bladder function. Because the nerves in the bladder that control urination are autonomic, diabetics with autonomic neuropathy may have problems emptying the bladder, compelling them to urinate often, to get up frequently during the night to urinate, or to suffer inadvertent leakage of urine (incontinence). Difficulty in completely emptying the bladder increases the risk of bladder infection. In some cases, the urine may travel back up into the kidneys, causing kidney problems.

Gastrointestinal Problems

High blood glucose may damage the autonomic nerves to the stomach and small and large intestines, causing gastrointestinal problems. When this happens, several scenarios may occur. Some people develop severe constipation; others, recurring diarrhea. Still others get a condition called gastroparesis, in which the stomach doesn't empty properly; they feel quite full after eating small amounts, and the sensation lasts several hours. Many people with this condition get diarrhea soon after the bloated feeling passes.

Managing Neuropathy

Prevention is the best approach to dealing with neuropathy. If you have diabetes, you can reduce your risk of developing neuropathy by as much as 60 percent by rigorously controlling your blood-sugar levels.

If you have painful neuropathy, your doctor may prescribe medicines to alleviate the pain. Men with poor erectile quality may benefit from medications or from other methods that treat impotence, such as using a vacuum device before intercourse or having a surgical implant. Women can use special lubricants to combat vaginal dryness.

If you have damage to the autonomic nerves, medicines can help you treat digestive problems or diarrhea. You can deal with some bladder problems by training yourself to urinate every few hours rather than waiting for the urge to go. Work with your health care team to deal with the problems that neuropathy can cause.

Kidney Problems

Diabetes accounts for about 40 percent of all instances of kidney failure, mostly in people with type 1 diabetes. High blood pressure further increases your chances of developing kidney failure and can make it worse.

By carefully controlling blood-glucose levels, the DCCT showed, people with type 1 diabetes can cut their risk of kidney disease in half.

The kidneys filter toxins and other wastes from the blood and flush them out of the body in the urine. At the same time, the kidneys allow the body to retain important proteins and other substances.

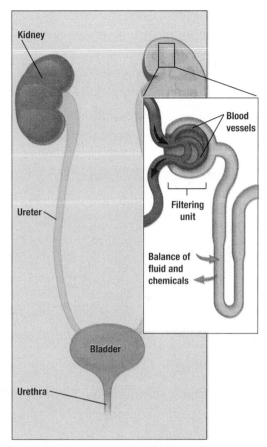

Kidney

Blood
vessels

Ureter

Filtering
unit

Balance of
fluid and
chemicals

Bladder

Urethra

> Kidneys filter toxins from the blood and
flush them from the body as urine.

A complex network of tiny blood vessels called glomeruli performs this filtering. Over time, high blood-glucose levels can damage the glomeruli, causing them to thicken and become distorted. As the damage worsens, the kidneys struggle to filter out wastes; proteins then begin to leak from the damaged blood vessels and into the urine.

One of the first signs of diabetic kidney disease is high levels of a protein called albumin in the urine. Everyone has small amounts of albumin in the urine, but higher levels than normal constitute a condition known as microalbuminuria. Over a period of 10 to 15 years, these albumin levels can steadily increase, indicating worsening kidney disease.

Kidney disease can creep up on you without symptoms. The reason: Healthy kidneys have about 10 times the capacity they need to do their filtering job. Therefore, most kidney problems do not typically show up until 90 percent of kidney function has been lost. When this happens, the body begins to retain fluid and salt, causing edema (swelling) in the hands and feet. The failure to rid the body of excess water and salt causes high blood pressure—or, if you already have high blood pressure, makes it worse. As kidney disease progresses, toxins accumulate in the body; you may experience nausea, fatigue, vomiting, loss of appetite, weakness, or itching. At this point, kidney disease is life-threatening, necessitating either dialysis or a kidney transplant.

Diagnosis and Treatment

As part of your regular checkups, your health care provider will perform urine and blood tests to gauge your albumin levels and measure the function of your kidneys. If the test results are abnormal, the doctor may order extra tests to ascertain whether your kidneys are working normally.

Keeping your blood-glucose levels as close to normal as possible is the first step in preventing kidney disease. Controlling blood pressure is critical too, for it can slow the progression of kidney disease in both type 2 and type 1 diabetes. If you have kidney disease, you may need to carefully monitor your protein intake to retard the disease and delay the need for dialysis or a kidney transplant. (You may also need to reduce the dosage of certain medications—or avoid them altogether.)

Your educator or dietitian will help you devise a good low-protein meal plan. Quitting smoking and maintaining good cholesterol levels can help as well.

Eye Problems

If you have diabetes of any type, you are at increased risk for certain eye diseases. These include diabetic retinopathy, a condition that occurs when high blood-sugar levels damage blood vessels inside the eye; glaucoma, in which pressure builds up in the eye and can degrade peripheral (side) vision; and cataracts, a clouding of the lens that focuses light in the eye. Knowing about these diseases can help you recognize their symptoms and manage them.

Diabetic Retinopathy

Diabetic retinopathy is a disease in which high blood-glucose levels damage blood vessels in an area in the back of the eye called the retina. The Diabetes Control and Complications Trial showed that people with diabetes who succeed in keeping their blood-sugar levels near normal can reduce their risk of retinopathy and other eye diseases by a staggering 76 percent.

Retinopathy occurs in two stages. In the first or nonproliferative stage, the walls of the blood vessels in the retina weaken and begin to leak fluid into the eye. This fluid deposits fat and proteins in the eye tissue. The blood vessels also develop tiny aneurysms (bulges) that leak blood into the retina. As the condition gets worse, the blood vessels begin to close, robbing the retina of its blood supply. Without a blood supply, nerves die off and white, cottony patches grow. If these patches are near the macula—the part of the retina that creates clear, sharp vision—your sight will deteriorate.

In the second or proliferative stage of retinopathy, the damaged retina tries to repair itself by growing fragile new blood vessels. But these

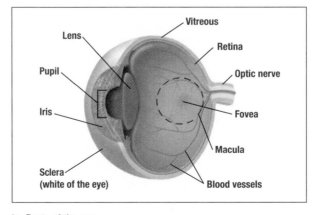

> Parts of the eye

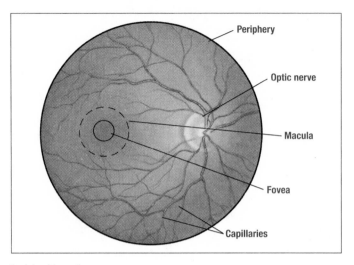

Periphery

Optic nerve

Macula

Fovea

Capillaries

> A healthy retina

new vessels are abnormal and grow into the compartment of the eye in front of the retina called the vitreous humor. Because they are fragile, they leak blood into the vitreous humor, which blocks light. This causes vision loss. As this blood is absorbed, the light can again pass through to the retina, but scar tissue forms. The scar tissue can attach itself to the retina and pull it away from the eye, resulting in a detached retina. This can lead to permanent vision loss. The proliferative stage is more common in people who have had diabetic retinopathy for a long time.

At first, diabetic retinopathy may cause neither eyesight problems nor other symptoms. As it progresses, however, seeing clearly may get harder. Some people see wavy lines. Vision may slowly worsen over time, or it may deteriorate quickly and without warning.

For all these reasons, regular eye examinations are of paramount importance for people with diabetes: Early detection is the key to preventing vision loss or blindness from diabetic retinopathy.

Symptoms of diabetic retinopathy may include:

• Having blurry, darkened, or cloudy vision
• Seeing floaters (dark spots) or black lines

Aggravating conditions. High blood pressure, high cholesterol, and smoking all exacerbate diabetic retinopathy. Pregnancy can aggravate it, too. Women with diabetes who become pregnant should have their eyes checked during pregnancy, especially during the first trimester. If possible, have your eyes examined before you get pregnant.

Detection. Schedule a complete eye exam at least once a year. The doctor can examine the deep interior of your eye to detect damage to retinal blood vessels before they have a chance to erode your vision. The doctor uses an eye chart and other tools to check your vision. He or she may use eye drops to dilate (widen) your pupils, permitting an inspection of your eyes for signs of disease. Here are some additional tests the doctor may perform:

- Tonometry, which measures fluid pressure inside the eye.
- Slit lamp exam, which lets the doctor view eye structures.
- Ultrasound, which uses sound waves to create an image of the eye. This test may be employed if blood is present in the vitreous humor (the "vitreous," for short).
- Fluorescein angiography, which uses special photographs of the retina to reveal even slight changes in capillaries in the eye. The photographs are used to document the amount of damage and track it over time.

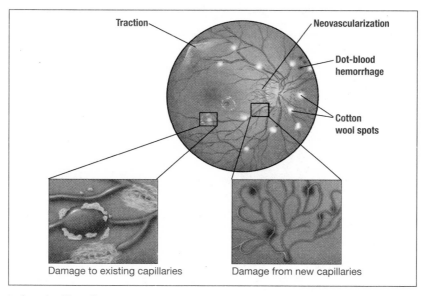

> An unhealthy retina

Treatment. If you have diabetic retinopathy, your eye doctor will design a treatment plan that's best for you. Early cases often do not need any treatment except good control of blood-glucose levels. Here are some customary treatments for diabetic retinopathy:

- Laser photocoagulation (to control leaking capillaries and prevent the growth of new capillaries)
- Vitrectomy (to remove a cloudy vitreous and scar tissue)
- Cryotherapy (to shrink capillaries and repair the retina)

Laser photocoagulation uses a laser beam (a high-energy light source) to treat diabetic retinopathy. The beam is focused on the retina, sealing weak capillaries and slowing the growth of new ones. Although this procedure does not cure diabetic retinopathy, it helps slow or halt the progress of the disease.

The type of treatment you receive depends on the extent and location of damaged capillaries. Treatment may take from a few minutes to half an hour or so. You may need more than one treatment session or type of treatment.

If the vitreous is clouded with blood, laser treatment must be deferred until the blood clears. If this is the case, **cryotherapy**—freezing the retina—may be used to shrink the abnormal blood vessels in the eye.

If blood or debris in the vitreous is clouding your vision or if your retina threatens to become detached, your doctor may recommend **vitrectomy.** This surgery uses tiny instruments to make small incisions in the eye, remove the cloudy vitreous, and replace it with fluid or gas. The surgery may take several hours.

Glaucoma

Glaucoma is an eye disease in which pressure builds up in the fluid inside the eyeball. This increase in fluid pressure damages the optic nerve, causing vision loss and even blindness. People can develop glaucoma whether they have diabetes or not, but people with diabetes get this eye disease more often and at a younger age.

In its early stages, glaucoma has no symptoms at all. You may have no way of knowing there is increased fluid pressure in your eyes, yet all the while that pressure is damaging your optic nerve. When symptoms begin, vision at the edges (periphery) is lost, causing tunnel vision.

During your regular eye examination, your doctor tests the pressure in your eyes and your peripheral vision—that is, how well and how far you can see to either side while looking straight ahead. If the fluid pressure is elevated, glaucoma can be treated with eye drops—and, in some cases, with laser surgery—to increase fluid drainage and reduce pressure.

Cataracts

Cataracts are a disease in which the eye's crystalline lens clouds over. Many people who do not have diabetes get cataracts, but people with diabetes often get them at a younger age.

Cataracts grow slowly and painlessly. Your eye doctor may discover early cataracts during your annual eye examination or you may notice some symptoms, such as a blurring or dimming of your vision or a new-found sensitivity to glare and lights.

Your eye doctor can treat your cataracts and restore the clarity of your vision. Normally, cataracts are not treated until they begin to interfere with everyday activities. The doctor performs surgery to remove the cataract and generally implants an intraocular lens—something like a hard contact lens—inside the eye.

Mouth Infections

If you have diabetes, you are more likely to get periodontal disease—that is, infections of the gum and tissues that support the teeth. Preventing periodontal disease requires ongoing dental care. Tell your dentist if you have any problems controlling your blood sugar; this alerts him or her to be hypervigilant for signs of periodontal disease.

What causes gum infections? Bacteria in your mouth form a sticky, whitish film, called plaque, on your teeth. If plaque is not removed daily, it can harden into a rough yellow or brown deposit called tartar; this is harder to remove from your teeth than plaque. Bacteria from plaque and tartar can cause swollen, infected, and receding gums as well as periodontal disease.

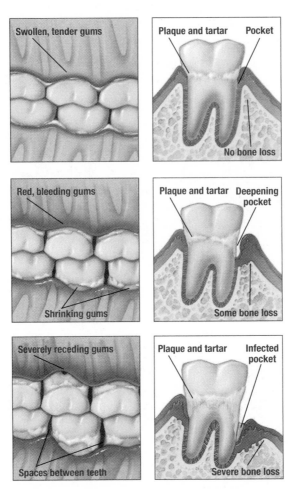

> Periodontal disease is more likely to occur if you have diabetes.

If you have periodontal disease, your dentist may want to see you every three to four months for exams and cleanings. The frequency of your visits will hinge on the severity of your disease. It may also depend on your plaque and tartar buildup, and on how well you care for your teeth and gums.

To control periodontal disease, your dentist may employ scaling and root planing to remove plaque and tartar from teeth above and below the gum line. You may need follow-up visits every three to four months to make sure your gum problem is under control. Additionally, your dentist may prescribe antibiotics—medications that kill bacteria—to treat periodontal disease. These may be in pill or topical form (that is, to be applied to a specific area).

If you have advanced periodontal disease or if the infection is not responding to other types of treatments, your dentist may perform gum surgery. This treatment method is designed to remove deep or unusually stubborn deposits of plaque and tartar.

Good oral hygiene can help avert periodontal disease. Brush your teeth (and your tongue) after every meal and floss at least once a day. Many doctors recommend a type of electric toothbrush that employs sonic waves because they believe it cleans better at the gum line. Anyone with diabetes should go for a dental cleaning at least once every six months. Keeping your blood glucose at a healthy level will help your body fight infections; such maintenance may also lessen the severity of periodontal disease.

Foot Problems

People with diabetes need to take extra-good care of their feet, especially if you have peripheral nerve damage and poor circulation from peripheral artery disease. If you do, even a small foot problem can become very serious. By working with a podiatrist (a specially trained foot doctor), you can learn how to protect your feet from damage and keep them healthy.

Neuropathy is especially vexing for people with diabetes because the loss of feeling caused by the disorder may make you unaware of injuries or sore spots on your feet. If you also have peripheral artery disease, it is harder for small problems, such as a blister, to heal properly. In fact, minor injuries—even an annoyance as seemingly simple as an ingrown toenail—can quickly become serious infections that send you to the hospital. Severe infections can lead to amputations.

Most foot problems are caused by rubbing or pressure in areas where skin lies close to bone. Although these problems can beset anyone, having high blood glucose makes them much more serious. If not treated, even a tiny break in the skin can become a severe infection. In

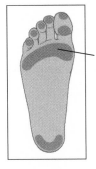

Pressure spots on the bottom of the foot absorb pressure from the body's weight. These are common areas in which problems can develop.

some cases, bones and joints can become infected from the skin without your knowing it.

Here are some common foot problems and their causes:

• Corns and calluses are the result of too much rubbing in the same spot. Over time, an infection may develop.

• Bunions result when the big toe is pushed inward, making the joint stick out. The bunion can get sore or infected. It may even evolve into arthritis.

• Ingrown toenails develop when the nail grows into the skin. This can let bacteria enter and lead to infections.

• A hammer toe is bent downward like a claw. This can create a corn or a blister where the joint sticks up on the top of the toe, or a blister where the toe tip rubs against the shoe.

All these foot problems easily lead to infection. Poor circulation can then inhibit healing, in which case the infection may spread. An infection may reach all the way through the skin and underlying tissues, spreading even to your joints or bones.

Preventing Foot Problems

If you have diabetes, the first step in preventing foot problems is to inspect your feet every day. This helps you find small skin irritations before they become serious infections. If you have trouble checking your feet, ask a family member or a friend to help. See your podiatrist right away if you have any of these problems:

> Common Foot Problems

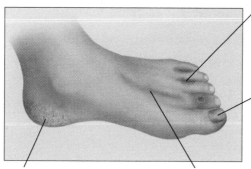

Athlete's Foot
Look for redness, scaling, or cracks around and between toes. This can be a sign of a fungal infection that causes itching and breaks in the skin.

Toenail Problems
Look for toenails growing into the skin and causing redness or pain. Thick, yellow, or discolored nails can signal a fungal infection.

Cracks in the Skin
Look for cracks on the heel and on the top and bottom of the foot. These are often caused by dry or irritated skin.

Color Changes
Look for any color changes in the foot. Redness with streaks can signal a severe infection, which needs immediate medical attention.

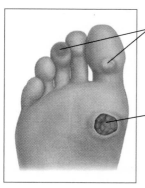

Hot Spots
Look for red "hot spots" in areas that get a lot of rubbing, such as the tops and bottoms of toes, the outer edge of the foot, and the ball of the foot. Over time, hot spots may turn into blisters, corns, calluses, or sores.

Sores, Ulcers, and Wounds
Look for sores in places such as the bottom of the big toe or the ball of the foot. Sores can have white, yellow, or clear drainage. See your podiatrist immediately if you have a sore.

- Red spots or blisters, corns, or calluses
- Drainage on your sock
- Dry, cracked, or scaly skin
- Thick, yellow, ingrown, or overly long toenails
- Slow-healing sores
- A tingling, cold, or burning sensation
- Numbness
- Red streaks or changes in skin color

It helps to check your feet at the same time every day so that the procedure becomes routine. Here's how to conduct a complete self-exam:

• Check the top of each foot. The tops of toes, the back of the heel, and the outer edge of the foot can get a lot of rubbing from poor-fitting shoes.

• Check the bottom of each foot. Daily wear and tear often leads to problems at pressure spots. If necessary, use a mirror to inspect the bottoms of your feet.

• Check the toes and nails. Fungal infections often occur between toes. Toenail problems can signal fungal infections or can lead to breaks in the skin.

• Check your shoes. Loose objects inside a shoe can injure your feet. Feel inside your shoes with your hand for potential irritants such as pebbles, loose stitching, or rough areas.

Practice these elements of good self-care to prevent foot problems:

• Manage your diabetes: Monitor and control your blood sugar, take medications as prescribed, eat healthy foods, and see your diabetes health care team members for regular checkups.

• Inspect your feet daily for hot spots, blisters, cracks, or dry skin.

• Avoid walking barefoot, even indoors. Always wear shoes and socks when not in bed. If you go swimming, wear swim shoes.

• Don't use corn or wart removers. These products often contain acid. Hydrogen peroxide can also make problems worse.

• Wash feet with warm water and mild soap every day. Don't soak your feet. Dry your feet well, especially between the toes.

• Don't trim corns, calluses, or toenails yourself. See your podiatrist for regular foot care and pedicures.

• Avoid tight stockings, socks, or pantyhose, all of which can restrict blood flow to your feet. Avoid sitting with your legs crossed for long stretches of time.

• Don't use heating pads on your feet. If you have neuropathy, you could get a burn and not feel it.

• If you smoke, stop now. Smoking restricts blood flow and can make it harder for wounds to heal.

Working with Your Podiatrist

A podiatrist is a health professional (but not a medical doctor) who specializes in treating the feet. He or she is therefore an essential member of the health care team for people with diabetes. When you visit your podiatrist, he or she will take a medical history, check the condition of your feet, and perhaps perform other tests.

As part of the examination, the podiatrist will check the nerves in your feet and assess the circulation in your extremities by taking a pulse in your feet. Your podiatrist will then develop a foot-care program for you, instructing you how to take special care of the feet. By remembering to check your feet daily—and by seeking immediate care from your podiatrist at the first sign of any problems—you should be able to keep your feet healthy for miles to come.

12

Lifestyle Considerations

Dealing with diabetes has never been easy. No matter how much you learn about how to manage the disease—and no matter how hard you work to lead a normal, healthy life—the condition can sometimes seem overwhelming. Managing your diet, making certain you get enough exercise, monitoring your blood glucose, taking your medication—all these are only a part of your daily routine.

So if simultaneously juggling everything you have to do and managing a chronic disease seems more than you can handle some days, give yourself a break. Call a friend and go to a movie. Treat yourself to a new book and hole up in your living room and read. Go fishing. In short, treat yourself to something you enjoy but rarely get to do.

One thing you should be aware of, however, is that stress and depression can affect more than just your mood. They can also affect your diabetes.

This chapter explains how and why dealing with the emotional side of diabetes does not substantially differ from learning how to deal with any physiological aspect of the disease. The three main steps in the process are to understand what's going on, learn to recognize the warning signs, and treat the problem.

When Stress Saps Your Strength

Stress comes in doses large and small, from losing your job to getting stuck in traffic or on public transport. On top of that, of course, is the continuing stress of living with diabetes day in and day out. No one needs to tell you how these various stressors affect your emotional health. You can feel them right away. You may get headaches, or you may act tense or grouchy with the people around you.

What you may not be able to see is the way such stress affects your physical health. When faced with stress, the body undergoes a "fight-or-flight" response designed to give you enough energy to deal with the situation at hand. The body releases energy stores (including glucose) and hormones (including insulin) that help your cells absorb the extra glucose. Diabetes upsets the balance: Glucose is released but insulin is not produced. Indeed, in people with type 2 diabetes, stress suppresses rather than spurs the release of insulin. As a result, blood-sugar levels tend to rise too high.

Whether they have diabetes or not, people may experience a range of other unhealthy reactions to stress. Under stress, they may:

• Exercise less, drink too much alcohol, or eat the wrong foods
• Run a higher risk of getting an infection
• Be likelier to suffer depression or anxiety

Strategies for Shrinking Stress

Try the following techniques to reduce stress or help you cope with it:

• Practice a relaxation technique, such as deep breathing, so it becomes a habit and you can draw on this technique during stressful moments.
• Limit or avoid alcohol and caffeine. (Remember that many soft drinks—even non-cola ones—contain caffeine.)
• Think of a stressful event as a challenge to be overcome. For instance, how might you change your work situation to make it less stressful?
• If you can't change a stressful situation, change your reaction to it. If you've just switched grocery lines only to find your original line wound up moving faster, for example, focus on staying calm. Rather than getting upset, use the time to practice deep breathing or page through a magazine.
• Take five to 10 minutes each day to sit, close your eyes, and allow your body tension to ease.

A Bad Mood—or Something More?

Psychologists catalog anxiety and depression as mood disorders, but suffering from either one is much more complex than a simple case of being in a bad mood.

Anxiety Disorder

Everyone occasionally feels worried or on edge, right? So when does anxiety cross the line from mere distraction to full-blown disorder?

Most instances of anxiety are perfectly normal. If your children are late getting home, for example, you may worry that they've been in an accident. If you're preparing to take a test or to be interviewed for a job, you're likely to feel anxious about doing well. Or perhaps your blood-glucose levels have been running a little high and you're concerned about your health. Occasional anxiety is part of life. As a matter of fact, small doses of the stuff may even be good for you: It keeps you on your toes, alert to danger, and primed to perform well. But if you find yourself feeling anxious and worried most of the time, especially with no apparent cause, you may be suffering from an anxiety disorder.

Do you find yourself constantly feeling as though something bad is about to happen, dreading everyday situations, or feeling tense and worried even when there is little or nothing to provoke these feelings? Think about the past six months. If you have been feeling anxious and tense for no apparent reason frequently, you may be suffering from an anxiety disorder.

An anxiety disorder may also produce physical symptoms, such as headaches, muscle tension and aches, fatigue, trembling, twitching, sweating, and irritability.

Feeling anxious occasionally may be perfectly normal, but feeling that way frequently is not. So talk to your doctor about treatments that can help you feel better.

Treatment options. Anxiety disorders often respond to psychotherapy or "talk" therapy. Two types of psychotherapy that seem to be particularly helpful for anxiety disorders are behavioral therapy and cognitive-behavioral therapy. Behavioral therapy involves working on changing certain actions and uses various techniques to stop unwanted behaviors. Cognitive-behavioral therapy teaches you to understand your thinking patterns and to change them so that you can change the way you react to situations that cause you anxiety.

Several medications can also help. Your doctor can prescribe a medication to help you with your anxiety or may refer you to a specialist who can. Certain medicines for treating anxiety take several weeks to kick in, so don't get discouraged if you don't feel better right away. Your doctor may also suggest a combination of medication and psychotherapy.

A Significant Sadness

Feeling depressed most of the time transcends mere moodiness. It is an illness called depression—a serious condition that affects your thoughts, feelings, and ability to function in everyday life.

How do you know if you or someone you know is suffering from depression? According to the National Institute of Mental Health, these are some of the symptoms:

- Persistent sad, anxious, or "empty" mood
- Feelings of hopelessness
- Feelings of guilt, worthlessness, or helplessness
- Loss of interest or pleasure in hobbies and activities you once enjoyed
- Loss of interest in sex
- Fatigue or decreased energy
- Trouble concentrating, remembering, or making decisions
- Sleep disturbances such as insomnia, waking too early, or sleeping too much
- Changes in appetite or weight (or both)
- Restlessness or irritability
- Thoughts of death or suicide attempts

If you experience five or more of these symptoms every day for at least two weeks—and if these symptoms interfere with your daily activities such as school, work, social life, or child care—you may be suffering from depression. To find out for certain, consult your health care provider.

Predisposed to depression? Although anyone can suffer from depression (and at any age), people with diabetes may have double the risk of the general population. First of all, many researchers believe that depression is the result of stress—and the difficulty of managing a chronic disease definitely qualifies as stress. Second, some researchers believe that the metabolic changes that occur in diabetes affect brain function in ways that cause depression.

Depression also seems to increase the risk of diabetic complications. This may be because it saps the energy you need to manage your diabetes. If you're depressed, you may be less likely to take care of yourself, to take your medication regularly, to exercise, or to follow your diet, any of which can make your diabetes worse. In a proverbial vicious circle, high blood-glucose levels worsen depression, and depression can make it harder to control your blood-glucose levels.

Whether diabetes causes depression or depression constitutes a risk factor for diabetes, getting treatment is critical. Above all, treatment will make you feel better. And if you feel better, you'll be likelier to take care of yourself. Instead of being trapped in the spiral of declining mental and physical health caused by depression, you'll embark upon a self-reinforcing process of positive behavior and improved well-being.

Treatment options. Your health care provider can help you with treatment for depression. She or he may refer you to a specialist: a psychologist, a psychiatrist, or a clinical social worker, any of whom can help you with counseling or "talk" therapy. Several antidepressant medications are available for treating depression; your doctor may prescribe one of these alone or in combination with counseling. This dovetailing of psychotherapy and medicine works especially well for most people.

Above all else, don't delay in seeking treatment for depression. The sooner you feel better, the better you'll care for yourself—and the more manageable your diabetes will become.

Diabetes and Sexual Problems

A husband recently diagnosed with diabetes told his wife, "There goes our sex life." Refusing to buy into this common myth, she insisted instead that they get up-to-date information about how to prevent—and, if called for, to treat—any sexual problems that may occur with diabetes. What they discovered is that diabetes-related problems may diminish arousal and orgasm. More often, however, sexual problems have their root cause in changes that occur in people's psyches, not bodies. A standard complication for men with diabetes is erectile dysfunction, often called ED. As explained in chapter 11, poorly controlled blood-glucose levels can cause nerve damage and vascular disease. The combined effect of the two conditions is to make men with diabetes three times as likely to experience ED as men without the disease. These problems may begin 10 to 15 years earlier than in men without diabetes.

Another sexual problem experienced by some men with diabetes is retrograde ejaculation. In this condition, part or all of a man's semen goes into the bladder rather than out of the penis during ejaculation. This happens when internal muscles called sphincters do not function normally—the result of nerve damage from poor blood-glucose control. As a consequence, the semen passes out of the penis not during orgasm but instead later on, mixed with urine. Though retrograde ejaculation is not harmful, it can impair fertility.

Men with diabetes may also have low testosterone levels. Low testosterone accounts for about five percent of diminished desire or erectile difficulties in the general population, but men with diabetes are especially susceptible to the deficit. So there's no question that it's worthwhile to have your hormone levels checked.

Men with diabetes may become less interested in sex. This change usually occurs in men with ED. Anxiety about sexual performance can lead to this loss of interest. And men who are depressed or who take certain medications (especially some heart and blood-pressure medications, but others, too) may lose interest in sex.

Some men with diabetes have trouble reaching orgasm. This problem may be caused by nerve or blood-vessel damage or by the inability to develop an adequate erection. Again, certain medications may trigger or intensify the problem.

Women with diabetes may experience problems with sexual function too. Vaginal dryness (that is, lack of lubrication) when aroused is a common result of poorly controlled blood-glucose levels, damage to nerves and blood vessels, or low levels of the female hormone estrogen. This can create discomfort during sexual intercourse, thus decreasing sexual response or desire. And because arousal results from vasocongestion (the flooding of blood vessels) in the genital region, women may also feel less of a sensation of fullness or arousal during sexual activity. Up to 35 percent of women with diabetes may have problems with sexual response: decreased desire for sex, inability to become or remain aroused, lack of sensation, or inability to reach orgasm.

Both men and women with diabetes have more frequent urinary-tract infections (UTIs) and yeast infections. If this occurs, health care providers suggest abstaining from intercourse until the infection clears up. At such times, many couples report, they simply switch their focus to sensual massage or manual stimulation of genitals (variety being the spice of life). Orgasm is usually not affected by the presence of a yeast infection or UTI. Indeed, sex therapists encourage all couples to think of intercourse as only one of many pleasurable ways that a couple can enjoy sexual activity together. Most find ways to increase sensory awareness and arousal. Sometimes practice with a new position, or the use of a vibrator, can increase sensory stimulation as well. Couples who include massage and manual stimulation as part of their regular sexual life, surveys show, tend to be more sexually active overall.

Because sexual response involves blood flow and the nervous system, certain blood-pressure drugs, antidepressants, and tranquilizers can cause sexual dysfunction as well. Many people report that they must learn to work with what is "normal" for them once they go on medications. In addition, 9 times out of 10 a doctor can make an appropriate medication change; to do so, however, he or she will need to know about the change in sexual function, so by all means speak up. And remember that both alcohol and tobacco aggravate sexual difficulties: They constrict the blood vessels that increase arousal.

In sex as in the rest of life, what happens in your head will affect your physical responses. Identify any emotional challenges that may be contributing to sexual problems. Stress, anxiety, and depression—all of which can easily befall people with diabetes—may hinder sexual enjoyment. Spectatoring—that is, overthinking your sexual responses—may make a mild sexual difficulty more problematic. Try to stay focused on the good feelings of skin on skin and the pleasure of enjoying your partner rather than judging your "performance" (an unfortunate word) in your head.

In this way, people with diabetes are just like everyone else: When you treat root causes, you confer a double benefit, simultaneously relieving an emotional condition and improving your sex life. Remember that we live in an age when medication or counseling (or a pairing of the two) can help.

So back to that myth of the vanishing love life: Though diabetes does not mean the end of sex, allowing yourself to think that way may constitute a self-fulfilling prophecy, leading you to experience problems that lack any true physical cause. Sexual problems are often psychological. From a medical standpoint, it is ordinarily many years before nerve damage or circulation problems reach the point where they interfere with sexual functioning. And even when problems do occur, effective treatments are often available.

Don't Ignore the Problem—Treat It

Sexual problems that stem from diabetes can often be treated. As with any sexual difficulty, the first step on the road to a solution is to acknowledge the problem. You and your partner can then take action to correct or accommodate that trouble.

High blood-glucose levels reduce sexual desire, so the better you control your diabetes the less it will erode your interest in sex. In addition, certain treatments can improve sexual functioning. For men, a number of prescription medications, mechanical devices, and surgical implants are available that can improve erectile quality. If testosterone levels are low, your doctor may recommend replacement with oral drugs, hormone shots, or gels or patches applied to the skin.

Women with vaginal dryness can use lubricants or topical estrogen for the vagina. If they have gone through menopause, they can ask their doctor about hormone replacement therapy (HRT), which may involve estrogen or testosterone. Not much research has been conducted on medically improving low libido or sexual response in women with diabetes (or in women in general, for that matter). But stay tuned. This is truly a "hot" topic, and sexologists believe that additional medications will be developed. In the meantime, focus on adapting to your body's changes to maximize pleasure. Find the time of day when you are rested and interested. Attend to your own needs and tune out distractions.

Many people are reluctant to talk about their sex lives. But treating a sexual dysfunction is a key part of managing your diabetes and a cornerstone of caring for your health and well-being. So if there's a problem, don't dismiss it—discuss it. Talk to your doctor about which treatments may be available—and appropriate—for you. If you have recently started a new medicine, explore whether it could be part of your problem.

Educating Others

With more than 21 million U.S. residents living with diabetes, you might assume the rest of the population would know a good deal—or at least something—about the disease. Not so. Chances are, you'll have to spend a fair amount of time educating your family and friends about what it means to have diabetes—and how, if at all, it will affect your time together.

Of course, your family will likely be more affected by your diabetes than your friends simply because you share living quarters. Family members may see you monitoring your blood sugar and taking insulin injections or other diabetes medications; if you're working or playing together, they may be obliged to work these activities into their daily schedules. Don't forget your co-workers. You may need their help in case of an emergency.

Dinner as Usual—or Better

You'll be sharing meals with your family, so the foods you prepare (or those prepared for you) must conform to your diet. But a diabetic meal plan is a healthy diet, and that means it can be good for other family members as well. Not only that, but healthy meals need not be any harder to prepare—in fact, they are probably easier—than those not-so-healthy ones featuring high-fat sauces or heavy desserts.

You will doubtless have to deal with the food issue when dining with friends, either in their homes or in a restaurant. If you're invited to a friend's house for a meal, your host may ask in advance whether he or she should prepare any special foods. Or if you're selecting a restaurant, your friends may wonder if they must choose one with a menu tailored to people with diabetes. Your response can be the same in both instances: Explain that your diet can accommodate most foods—even desserts—so long as you take care to balance the foods you eat and closely monitor their quantities.

With careful attention, you should be able to join your friends for virtually any type of meal and still find foods to fit your diet. This will be easier with some meals than others, of course, so speak up whenever you realize a suggested menu or venue will pose problems.

Exercise

Exercise, that crucial commodity for all people with diabetes, is beneficial to those without the disease as well. Make it a family affair: Start off with a simple walk through the neighborhood, then work up to a hike in a wilderness area.

Setting Limits

You may find certain family members or friends occasionally getting a little too involved in your diabetes. They may tell you about a new "miracle" treatment they think you should try or instruct you what to eat or how to take your medication. Though well-intentioned, these efforts are misguided. You'll listen to their concerns, of course, but as you well know by now, managing your diabetes is ultimately your job and no one else's.

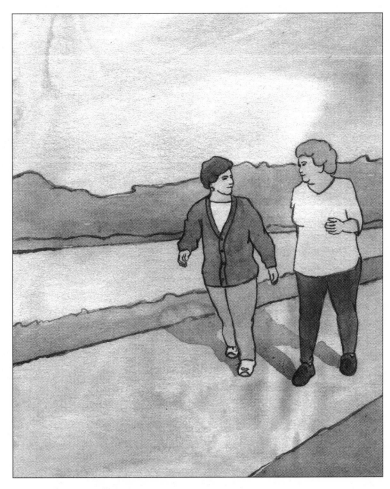

> Exercise is a boon to all—especially diabetics.

Your Lifestyle, Your Life

Armed with your newfound knowledge of how to cope with diabetes on a daily basis, you're aware that the disease need not keep you from leading an active, satisfying life. Granted, you must recognize your own limits, eat well, and exercise regularly. You need to tend constantly to your emotional and physical health, avoid stress, watch for signs of depression, and communicate openly with your partner, your family, your friends, and, to some extent, your co-workers.

Just remember that you're not in this alone. When you feel you need help with anything—whether it's managing blood-sugar levels or dealing with your diet or handling pressures at work or at home—remind yourself that you have a team of diabetes specialists trained to support you in managing the disease.

Which brings us to the last item you need to perform as regularly as you do everything else: Stop and give yourself a pat on the back for a job well done. Living with diabetes presents some uniquely thorny challenges, and you are meeting and dealing with them every day.

13 What's Ahead

Scientists, health care professionals, and educators now know a good deal about diabetes. They know how to diagnose it and how to manage it. They know a few ways to prevent type 2 diabetes and are searching for more. They also know how diabetes affects the body, how it progresses over time, and how to fend off some of its complications.

But several vital nuggets of knowledge continue to elude these experts: What goes wrong with insulin production and insulin resistance in type 2 diabetes? What causes the body's immune system to attack and kill insulin-producing cells in the pancreas in type 1? And, finally, is there a cure for diabetes? These vital questions have yet to be answered.

Is There a Cure?

Although diabetes has no pharmaceutical cure, a handful of treatments currently under study offer the possibility of a surgical cure. The three most promising are detailed below.

Pancreas Transplant

This type of surgery is performed to implant a healthy pancreas from a donor into a person with type 1 diabetes. The transplanted organ gives the person with diabetes a chance to cease taking insulin.

In a pancreas transplant, the patient's diseased pancreas is not removed; rather, the donor pancreas is inserted into the lower right side of the abdomen. A portion of the donor's duodenum (part of the intestine) is also transplanted to receive the digestive enzymes that the pancreas secretes besides insulin.

After a transplant, a person must take powerful drugs to suppress the immune system to keep it from rejecting the donor pancreas. It is the need for these medications that greatly limits the usefulness of this surgery.

If the person receiving the transplant also has kidney disease, a kidney transplant is often performed at the same time. Indeed, many hospitals refuse to perform a pancreas transplant unless the person needs a kidney as well. The reason: The drugs that suppress the immune system make the person susceptible to so many other diseases that the cure (the drugs) may be more dangerous than the disease (diabetes).

On the other hand, if a person is having a kidney transplant and will need these drugs anyway, most hospitals will consent to perform a pancreas transplant, if one is needed, as part of the same surgery.

Although pancreas transplant has been available as a diabetes treatment for more than 10 years, donor organs are scarce. Only about 1,300 of these operations are performed each year, but they have a solid success rate: From 83 to 94 percent of pancreas transplants are successful at three years after surgery, and 68 percent at 10 years, freeing the person from the need to take insulin. On the other hand, many recipients of pancreas transplants get sick from the immunosuppressant drugs, making this procedure an unsatisfactory option for most people.

Islet-Cell Transplant

Another surgical method, called an islet-cell transplant, is being studied for treating diabetes. In this procedure, only the islet portions of pancreatic cells (the site of insulin-producing beta cells) are transplanted.

An islet-cell transplant is simpler and less invasive than transplanting an entire pancreas into a diabetic patient. Healthy islets from a donor pancreas are purified, then introduced through a small tube into a vein in the liver. To forestall rejection of the transplanted cells, patients must take drugs to suppress their immune system for the rest of their lives. A successful islet-cell transplant can restore blood-sugar levels to normal without the need for insulin.

Islet-cell transplants remain in the experimental stages. As with pancreas transplants, the medications taken to suppress rejection can throw open the doors to many other problems. As such, islet-cell transplants are available only to people who participate in clinical studies. Not only that, but the shortage of donor pancreases limits the availability of islet cells for transplant.

Stem-Cell Transplants

Stem cells are cells in the body that have the potential to transform into several different specific kinds of cells, such as the beta cells of the pancreas. In the laboratory, these cells can be induced to transform themselves into cells with special functions—in which case they can be used to replace damaged cells. Scientists believe that stem cells hold great promise for treating people with diabetes, Parkinson's disease, heart disease, and birth defects. However, stem-cell research is controversial and is not available for use in humans at this time.

Improved Treatments

As research continues into a diabetes cure, improved treatments for the disease are constantly being developed.

New Ways to Deliver Insulin

Thanks to technological advances, more efficient ways to deliver insulin are becoming available. At one time, the only method for taking insulin was by injection, using a syringe. Nowadays, people who must take insulin can choose among the syringe, insulin pen, jet injector, insulin pump, and insulin inhaler. New developments, described below, may facilitate the delivery of insulin even more.

Implanted insulin pump. Research is under way on a special type of insulin pump that can be implanted under the skin in the abdomen and programmed to deliver insulin into the abdominal cavity or a large vein. The pump would eliminate the need for multiple daily insulin injections. The user would monitor blood glucose and use the pump's remote-control unit to tell the pump how much insulin to deliver. Participants in clinical studies of the implanted insulin pump showed better control of blood-glucose levels and fewer episodes of hypoglycemia than they had been able to achieve with external pumps or insulin injections. The implanted system controls blood sugar better than the current insulin pumps because it delivers insulin directly into a large vein rather than into the skin, where it is absorbed slowly.

Oral insulin. Insulin cannot be taken by mouth because the body's digestive acids attack and destroy the hormone before it has a chance to do its work. However, researchers are working on a polymer-coated pill that would shield the insulin from stomach enzymes. The insulin in the pill remains intact until the pill passes from the stomach to the intestine, where it can be absorbed. So far, this oral insulin has been tested only in animals. It must be studied more extensively before being tested in humans.

Insulin patch. Just as people wear a patch to deliver hormones, nicotine, or other medication through the skin, people who need insulin may someday be able to receive it from a patch. At this time, the patch can deliver only small doses of insulin. As research on it advances, however, the insulin patch may be perfected to deliver single or continuous doses as needed.

New Oral Medications

Scientists continue to study ways to improve medications to make the body less resistant to insulin and to stimulate insulin secretion. The growing body of scientific knowledge about the causes and effects of diabetes should steadily usher in new and refined medications to treat type 2. Indeed, new types of medication to treat diabetes are on the horizon.

Continuous Glucose Monitoring

The goal of research into blood-glucose monitoring has been to develop a system of continuous monitoring that will yield frequent, accurate readings. Such ongoing readings would be particularly helpful to diabetics at a high risk of severe hypoglycemia. Some continuous monitoring systems are now available, and new ones are in development.

Looking to the Future

Researchers are exploring ways to cure diabetes or improve its treatment. Someday they may hit upon methods not only to cure the disease, but also to prevent it. Until that day dawns, you should manage your diabetes with the best tools currently available: watching your diet, exercising, and wisely using medication to keep your blood-sugar levels as close to normal as possible.

APPENDIX A

Resources

The resources listed below provide links to web pages offering a panoply of useful information about diabetes and its treatment. All links were robust at press time; because web addresses change frequently, however, some links may be obsolete. If you encounter a nonfunctioning link, go to the organization's home page and use its search engine to locate the information.

General Information on Diabetes

American Diabetes Association (ADA)
www.diabetes.org
This website is one of the best online resources for information on every aspect of diabetes, including recipes and exercise advice. The ADA is a nonprofit health organization supporting diabetes re-search and providing information and advocacy. Its mission is "to prevent and cure diabetes and to improve the lives of all people affected by diabetes." ADA supports research, provides information and other services, and distributes scientific findings related to diabetes. The ADA also advocates for scientific research and for the rights of people with diabetes. It conducts programs in all 50 states and the District of Columbia, reaching hundreds of communities. The association's website provides links to activities in your area. Information is available in English and Spanish.

All about diabetes
www.diabetes.org/about-diabetes.jsp
This ADA web page provides an excellent overview of the disease and defines the major types of diabetes. It also provides information for

people recently diagnosed, a description of diabetes symptoms, some of the myths about diabetes, statistics, and an explanation of a diabetes health care team. You can also link to webcasts on several diabetes topics and access the Diabetes Learning Center, which provides information for people who have recently been diagnosed. There is also a link to a risk-assessment quiz.

Diabetes dictionary
www.diabetes.org/diabetesdictionary.jsp?WTLPromo=FOOTER _dictionary
An excellent and comprehensive online dictionary of diabetes terminology.

Are you at risk for obesity?
http://diabetes.org/weightloss-and-exercise/are-you-at-risk.jsp
Learn how to assess your risk for diabetes based on your body weight. This website also explains the value of weight loss and exercise and how these affect diabetes risk and diabetes management for those who have the disease. The website includes a calculator for body mass index, guidance on weight loss, meal-planning tips for dieters, and information on the role of exercise in preventing diabetes.

Diabetes prevention
www.diabetes.org/diabetes-prevention.jsp
Do you know what steps you can take to help prevent type 2 diabetes? This website describes them, including explanations of prediabetes, how to prevent or delay diabetes, and a diabetes-risk test.

Centers for Disease Control and Prevention (CDC)
http://www.cdc.gov/diabetes/consumer/
The CDC, a part of the U.S. Department of Health and Human Services, supports several programs that address chronic diseases such as diabetes. CDC's online resources are easy to access and are available in English, Spanish, and other languages. The CDC diabetes webpage guides consumers to information on virtually ever aspect of diabetes, from prevention to management.

What is diabetes?
www.cdc.gov/diabetes/pubs/pdf/prevent.pdf
This eight-page online booklet describes diabetes, who is at risk, symptoms, management, and how to prevent the disease. It is available in English and Spanish.

Basics about diabetes
www.cdc.gov/diabetes/faq/basics.htm
The compendium of diabetes information that originates on this webpage provides links to separate sections dealing with symptoms, types of diabetes, risk factors, treatment, and prevention.

Diabetes and me
www.cdc.gov/diabetes/consumer/prevent.htm
Are you one of the millions of Americans at risk for diabetes? This CDC website offers guidance for preventing diabetes through diet and exercise. It also presents risk-assessment tools. It is accessible in English and Spanish.

Medline plus
medlineplus.gov/
The National Library of Medicine and the National Institutes of Health operate this website. It provides consumer-friendly information on specific disease topics and conditions, as well as links to medical encyclopedias and dictionaries, drug information, directories of doctors and hospitals, and other resources. You can research diabetes information here as well as information on related conditions.

Juvenile Diabetes Research Foundation (JDRF)
www.jdrf.org
Although the JDRF conducts research and provides support and advocacy related to type 1 diabetes, much of the information it offers is relevant to people with type 2 diabetes. The webpage includes links to checklists for dealing with diabetic emergencies. The information is designed to inform people unfamiliar with the clinical aspects of diabetes what to do in case of a diabetes emergency in a friend or co-worker. The JDRF site also includes sample diabetes-care forms for schools.

National Diabetes Information Clearinghouse (NDIC)

www.diabetes.niddk.nih.gov/index.htm

The NDIC is an information-dissemination service of the National Institute of Diabetes and Digestive and Kidney Diseases (NIDDK), which in turn is part of the National Institutes of Health (NIH). NDIC and NIDDK are two of the richest online resources for people with diabetes. Their websites provide information that includes an overview of the disease, available treatments, complications and how to prevent them, diabetes statistics, clinical trials in diabetes, and other resources. The site is accessible in both English and Spanish.

Your guide to diabetes: Type 1 and type 2

www.diabetes.niddk.nih.gov/dm/pubs/type1and2/index.htm

This guide to managing diabetes includes links to information on managing diabetes under various circumstances, such as when your blood-glucose levels are too high or too low, daily diabetes management, and where to get help with your diabetes.

Diabetes dictionary

diabetes.niddk.nih.gov/dm/pubs/dictionary

Are you confused by the profusion of diabetes terminology? This website defines the key terms used when health care professionals and others discuss the disease.

Diagnosing diabetes

diabetes.niddk.nih.gov/dm/pubs/diagnosis/index.htm

This comprehensive source provides information on the diagnosis, prevention, and management of diabetes, with links to sections describing diabetes and prediabetes, how diabetes is diagnosed, risk factors, when to get tested, how to prevent or delay diabetes, and other vital information.

Monitoring Blood Glucose

Medline Plus: Blood-glucose monitoring
www.nlm.nih.gov/medlineplus/ency/article/003438.htm
Review the ABCs of glucose monitoring. This site explains the process of glucose monitoring step by step—including how the test is performed, normal and abnormal values, and more.

U.S. Food and Drug Administration (FDA)
www.fda.gov/
The FDA is the federal regulatory agency responsible for guaranteeing the safety of the nation's foodstuffs and medicines. Its website offers a wealth of information on diabetes medications and equipment.

Glucose meters & diabetes management
www.fda.gov/diabetes/glucose.html
This corner of the FDA website offers everything you need to know about blood-glucose monitoring. Included are monitoring devices, how to use glucose meters, choosing a meter, and factors that affect meter performance, as well as information on other diabetes-management tests.

National Diabetes Information Clearinghouse (NDIC)
Noninvasive Blood-Glucose Monitoring
diabetes.niddk.nih.gov/dm/pubs/glucosemonitor/index.htm

Diabetes Medications and Insulin
NDIC
Alternative devices for taking insulin
diabetes.niddk.nih.gov/dm/pubs/insulin/index.htm
This website describes alternatives to conventional syringe injections, including insulin pens, pumps, inhaled insulin, and subcutaneous infusion sets. It also discusses new delivery methods under development.

Specific medications
diabetes.niddk.nih.gov/dm/pubs/medicines_ez/specific.htm#
insulin

This website provides descriptions of specific diabetes medications and insulins with discussions of how they work, dosages, and possible side effects.

Medicines for people with diabetes
diabetes.niddk.nih.gov/dm/pubs/medicines_ez/printer
friendly.htm

Consult this website for a list of questions to ask your health care provider or pharmacist about your diabetes medication, as well as a form for you to fill in with the name and dosage of your medication, the normal range for your glucose levels, and notes about when you should contact your doctor.

Diet, Nutrition, and Diabetes

American Academy of Family Physicians (AAFP)
familydoctor.org/349.xml

This part of the AAFP website answers frequently asked questions about diabetes and nutrition, including an explanation of food exchanges with a table of sample exchanges. Information is available in English and Spanish.

ADA
Diabetes and the food pyramid: Alcohol
www.diabetes.org/nutrition-and-recipes/nutrition/alcohol.jsp

This simple, informative summary explains how to manage alcohol consumption if you drink and have diabetes. It covers how to mix food and alcohol and details why additional blood-glucose monitoring is necessary before and after alcohol consumption.

Diabetes and metabolic health

http://diabetes.org/weightloss-and-exercise/diabetes-metabolic-health.jsp

If you have diabetes, you are more likely to be overweight or obese, and more likely to have high blood pressure and high cholesterol. About 20 percent of people with diabetes have more than one metabolic problem at the same time. This puts them at risk for heart disease.

Healthy weight loss

www.diabetes.org/weightloss-and-exercise/weightloss-healthy-weight-loss.jsp

This site offers realistic advice for losing weight and keeping it off. It explains the pitfalls of crash diets and offers tips for making weight loss easier.

Nutrition & recipes

www.diabetes.org/nutrition-and-recipes/nutrition/overview.jsp

This website is one of the most comprehensive online sources of information about diet and diabetes. It explains how eating well-balanced meals in the correct amounts can help you keep your blood-glucose level as close to normal as possible. It also includes sections on choosing foods and reading food labels, and it offers recipes and tips for cooking and nutrition.

Recipe of the day

www.diabetes.org/home.jsp

Mediterranean stuffed zucchini, anyone? Whether you like to cook or not, it's fun to read the daily recipes posted by the ADA. These dishes are easy to prepare, good to eat, and healthful for people with diabetes. Look for the link on the association's home page that reads "Recipe of the Day."

Weight loss and exercise

www.diabetes.org/weightloss-and-exercise.jsp

This site describes how losing weight—and keeping it off—can improve your overall health and your diabetes. It also describes exercise and its importance to diabetes management.

CDC
Diabetes and me: Eat right
www.cdc.gov/diabetes/consumer/eatright.htm

This CDC website offers tips on healthy eating, weight control, recipes, and special diets. It also includes links to other good sources of guidance on eating well with diabetes. Information is available in English and Spanish.

NDIC
What I need to know about eating and diabetes
diabetes.niddk.nih.gov/dm/pubs/eating_ez/

In addition to information on diet and diabetes, this website includes sections on how exercise fits into an overall diabetes-management plan. It also provides information on how to deal with hypoglycemia and offers detailed guidance on food types and adhering to your diet during illness.

Exercise and Weight Control

ADA
Weight Loss Matters
www.diabetes.org/weightloss-and-exercise/weightloss.jsp

Weight Loss Matters is a program sponsored by the ADA to help people with diabetes lose weight and manage their disease. The website includes an overview of diabetes, information on how to assess your risk for obesity, getting started on a weight-management plan, and how to start and maintain an exercise program.

American Volkssport Association (AVA)
www.ava.org/

This association of walkers invites you to join its members across the United States in walking local scenic trails at your own pace for health, fitness, and fun. Each year, AVA's network of 350 walking clubs organizes more than 3,000 walking events in all 50 states. (There is also the occasional bike, ski, or swim.) All events are open to the public.

American Yoga Association
www.americanyogaassociation.org/

The American Yoga Association is a nonprofit educational organization that provides yoga instruction and educational resources to anyone interested in learning more about this exercise that combines the physical and the spiritual. It serves as a resource for yoga students and teachers who have questions and concerns. "Easy Does It Yoga" is a special program designed for older adults or the physically challenged.

CDC
Body Mass Index (BMI) Calculator
http://www.cdc.gov/nccdphp/dnpa/bmi/

This easy-to-use BMI calculator asks for your height in inches and weight in pounds, obviating the need to convert to metric measurements. That makes finding out where you stand, weight-wise, a mouse click away.

Growing Stronger: Strength Training for Older Adults
www.cdc.gov/nccdphp/dnpa/physical/growing_stronger/
growing_stronger.pdf

Growing Stronger is an exercise program based on scientific research involving exercises that have been proven to increase the strength of your muscles, maintain the integrity of your bones, and improve your balance, coordination, and mobility. (Strength training can also help reduce the signs and symptoms of many chronic diseases, including arthritis.) This website describes strengthening exercises step by step with full illustrations, including warm-up and cool-down routines.

Physical Activity for Everyone
How active do adults need to be?
www.cdc.gov/nccdphp/dnpa/physical/recommendations/
adults.htm

No matter what your age or ability, moderate-intensity physical activity is a vital component of a healthy lifestyle. This site describes the range of recommended physical activity, explaining how much exercise you should strive for and how to build up to it. Included is a table for assessing your physical activity, with recommendations on how to move up from your current level. The site also explains how physical activity can prevent and help treat many common chronic medical conditions.

National Heart, Lung, and Blood Institute
Guide to Physical Activity
www.nhlbi.nih.gov/health/public/heart/obesity/lose_wt/
phy_act.htm
Explains just what constitutes "moderate" exercise and the importance of daily physical activity.

Weight Control Information Network (WIN)
Tips to Help You Get Active
win.niddk.nih.gov/
WIN is a program of the National Institute of Diabetes and Digestive and Kidney Diseases (part of the NIH). This website presents information in a question-and-answer format to help you identify your own barriers to physical activity; it also suggests ways to overcome them. WIN offers an extensive list of free publications on integrating exercise into your lifestyle.

Alternative and Complementary Medicine
American Botanical Council
www.herbalgram.org
This online source of information on "herbal news" is sponsored by an independent, nonprofit organization that promotes the responsible use of herbal medicine.

American Association of Naturopathic Physicians
www.naturopathic.org
The American Association of Naturopathic Physicians is a national professional society that represents naturopathic physicians who are either licensed or eligible for licensing. It publishes information for the public on naturopathic medicine and its principles.

American Association of Oriental Medicine
www.aaom.org

If you are interested in the traditional Chinese medical treatment known as acupuncture, this is a great website for locating a qualified practitioner in your area. Representing American acupuncturists committed to high standards and a well-regulated profession, the American Association of Oriental Medicine works to protect the well-being of the public.

American Chiropractic Association
www.amerchiro.org

The American Chiropractic Association is the professional association representing doctors of chiropractic—a therapy based on the premise that disease results from a lack of normal nerve function. Chiropractors use manipulation and adjustments of body structures, such as the spine, to treat illness. This website provides links to help you locate a certified chiropractor in your area.

American Massage Therapy Association
www.amtamassage.org

This professional organization works to advance the profession through ethics and standards, certification, school accreditation, continuing education, publications, legislative efforts, public education, and member development. This website provides links for those interested in locating a certified massage therapist in their area.

Center for Mind-Body Medicine
www.cmbm.org

The Center for Mind-Body Medicine provides information for patients and health care professionals on how the mind and body interact with respect to illness and how such techniques as meditation, biofeedback, and guided imagery can improve health. The website also includes a state-by-state listing of certified mind-body practitioners.

National Center for Complementary and Alternative Medicine (NCCAM)
nccam.nih.gov
This NIH agency explores complementary and alternative medicine (CAM) healing practices within a rigorously scientific context. It trains CAM researchers and disseminates authoritative information to the public and professionals. This website is a good place to research the effectiveness of herbal supplements. You can also find information here on virtually any CAM therapy.

NCCAM's diabetes information
http://nccam.nih.gov/health/diabetes/
Use this web address to access NCCAM information that relates specifically to diabetes. But don't stop there. The NCCAM site includes updates about clinical trials and other crucial research that is best reached via its search feature (just type "diabetes" into the search box on NCCAM's home page, ncam.nih.gov).

National Library of Medicine, Medline Plus
www.nlm.nih.gov/medlineplus/herbalmedicine.html
This website provides an overview of, and the latest news on, herbal supplements. It is available in English and Spanish.

Short-Term and Long-Term Complications

ADA
Diabetes, Heart Disease, and Stroke
diabetes.org/diabetes-heart-disease-stroke.jsp
This website describes "Make the Link!"—a special joint initiative between the ADA and the American College of Cardiology. It explains the relationship among diabetes, cholesterol levels, and heart attack and stroke.

Hypoglycemia
www.diabetes.org/type-2-diabetes/hypoglycemia.jsp
Make your way here for an extensive discussion of hypoglycemia and how to treat it. The website includes a link to an online training video on using glucagon to treat hypoglycemia.

CDC
Diabetes-related health concerns
www.cdc.gov/DIABETES/faq/concerns.htm
Answers frequently asked questions about diabetes. These include the complications of diabetes, organ systems affected, sexuality issues, depression, and how to manage diabetes when you are ill.

NDIC
Hypoglycemia
diabetes.niddk.nih.gov/dm/pubs/hypoglycemia/index.htm
This resource describes the causes, symptoms, and treatments of hypoglycemia.

Complications
diabetes.niddk.nih.gov/complications/index.htm
Check this website for information on diabetes complications and how to prevent or treat them, as well as information on sexual and urologic problems associated with the disease.

Lifestyle Considerations

ADA
Depression and anxiety
www.diabetes.org/diabetes-research/summaries/depression.jsp
This central site links to discussions of anxiety, sexual dysfunction, stress management, and depression (including how high blood-glucose levels can worsen depression).

Traveling with diabetes supplies
http://diabetes.org/advocacy-and-
legalresources/discrimination/public_accommodation/travel.jsp
The ADA has been working with the Transportation Safety Administration in the wake of September 11 to ensure that people with diabetes can keep their equipment and medications in their carry-on luggage when they are screened for boarding a plane. This website offers an overview of regulations and gives advice for traveling with syringes, insulin, and glucose-monitoring equipment and supplies.

When you travel
www.diabetes.org/type-2-diabetes/travel.jsp
The ADA has developed comprehensive information and advice for travelers with diabetes. Check this website for guidance on packing insulin and other supplies, managing your diet on the road, and other critical aspects of travel.

AARP
www.aarp.org/usingmeds
Using Meds Wisely: A tip sheet available from this AARP website gives advice about traveling with medications, both for diabetes and for other conditions.

National Institute of Mental Health (NIMH)
www.nimh.nih.gov
NIMH, part of the NIH, provides information on emotional and mental disorders. These include anxiety disorders and depression, their symptoms, how to treat them, and resources for obtaining help locally.

Depression and diabetes
www.nimh.nih.gov/publicat/depdiabetes.cfm
This fact sheet summarizes what diabetes patients need to know about depression.

Advocacy and Legislation

The U.S. Equal Employment Opportunity Commission
www.eeoc.gov/facts/diabetes.html

Describes the Americans with Disabilities Act with information on the rights and responsibilities of applicants, employees, and employers as they relate to diabetes as a disability.

ADA
Health insurance in your state
http://diabetes.org/advocacy-and-legalresources/insurance/overview.jsp

Obtaining health insurance can be a daunting hurdle for people with diabetes. The ADA has assembled comprehensive information on health-insurance options in all 50 states. Click on your state and the site provides an overview of COBRA, Medicaid, and other insurance options.

NDIC
Financial help for diabetes care
diabetes.niddk.nih.gov/dm/pubs/financialhelp/index.htm

This website provides links to information on various forms of financial assistance for people with diabetes, including Medicare, Medicaid, State Children's Health Insurance Program, hospital care, regular health insurance, and managed care. It also lists resources for prescription drugs, medical supplies, and prosthetic care.

APPENDIX B

Managing Your Diabetes When You Are Sick

Illnesses that most people take in stride, such as a bout of stomach flu or a cold, can be serious for people with diabetes. This is because sickness upsets your normal routine for managing your diabetes. When you are sick, your blood-glucose levels may rise: As your body fights off the infection, it produces stress hormones, which counteract the glucose-regulating effects of insulin. And if your illness keeps you from eating normally, your blood-glucose levels may fall too low, causing hypoglycemia. Check with your doctor so you'll know in advance what special precautions to take if you get sick.

Here is some guidance for how to deal with illness if you have diabetes:

• Don't stop taking your diabetes medicine or insulin. This advice holds true even if you can't eat. Because illness can cause your blood-sugar levels to rise, your doctor may advise you to take more medicine when you are sick.

• Monitor your blood-glucose levels more frequently (ask your doctor how often to do so) and keep track of the results. This will allow you to detect high or low blood glucose and work with your doctor to remedy it.

• If your glucose is 240 mg/dL or higher, test your urine for ketones—chemicals the liver makes when not enough insulin is in the blood. Use ketone strips, which you can buy at the drugstore.

• If you have a fever, drink extra liquids. Try to drink at least 1/2 cup (4 ounces) to 3/4 cup (6 ounces) every 30 to 60 minutes, even if you have to do so one sip at a time. These liquids should not have calories. Water, caffeine-free diet soda, or tea without sugar, are good choices.

• Try to eat normally. If you can't eat your usual foods, eat soft foods and liquids containing the same amount of carbohydrates you normally consume. You can try drinking juice or eating crackers, popsicles, or soup.

• If you can't keep food down, drink a clear liquid containing sugar, such as ginger ale. You need the carbohydrates to reduce your risk of hypoglycemia.

• Check your temperature regularly every morning and every evening. If you have a fever, it could mean you have an infection.

If you experience any of the following symptoms, contact your doctor or someone on your health care team right away or go to an emergency room:

• You are too sick to eat normally and you go more than six hours without being able to keep food down.

• You have severe diarrhea or throw up more than once in six hours.

• Your temperature is over 101° F.

• Your blood glucose remains higher than 300 mg/dL.

• You have moderate or large amounts of ketones in your urine (indicated by a ketone test strip turning purple).

• You have trouble breathing or can't think clearly.

The Centers for Disease Control and Prevention developed the following chart to help people with diabetes substitute foods when they're feeling too ill to eat regularly. (Many diabetic diets are based on exchanges, which are lists of foods that have similar amounts of carbohydrate, protein, and fat. An exchange is a specific amount of a certain type of food. Food-exchange groups are generally divided into starch/breads, meats, vegetables, fruits, dairy products, and fats.)

What to Eat or Drink When You're Sick

(Each item equals one bread or fruit exchange*)

Food Item	Amount
Fruit juice	1/3 to 1/2 cup
Fruit-flavored drink	1/2 cup
Soda (regular, not diet)	1/2 cup
*Jell-O® (regular, not sugar-free)	1/2 cup
*Popsicle® (regular, not sugar-free)	1/2 twin
Sherbet	1/4 cup
Saltine crackers	6 squares
Milk	1 cup
Thin soup (examples: vegetable, chicken noodle)	1 cup
Thick soup (examples: cream of mushroom, tomato)	1/2 cup
Ice cream (vanilla)	1/2 cup
Pudding (sugar-free)	1/2 cup
Pudding (regular)	1/4 cup
Macaroni, noodles, rice, mashed potatoes	1/2 cup (cooked)

*Use of trade names is for identification only and does not imply endorsement by the U.S. Department of Health and Human Services or by AARP.
SOURCE: Centers for Disease Control and Prevention
www.cdc.gov/DIABETES/pubs/tcyd/ktrack.htm#care

Travel Tips

Talk to Your Health Care Provider

Before you take off on a trip, talk with your health care provider about how to time your medicine, food, and activity. Ask what to do if you find changes in your glucose readings.

Traveling to a different time zone? Remember to adjust your timing of food, medicine, and activity. Your health care provider can help you with this. In addition, ask about healthful food and drink choices.

If you're leaving the country, obtain a signed letter from your doctor stating that you have diabetes and that it is a medical requirement that you carry your medications or insulin with you. Some countries may demand such documentation upon entry. It's likewise a good idea to get your doctor to write a prescription for you to get additional insulin, medication, or supplies, if needed. Ask your doctor to include an e-mail contact if further follow-up is required.

Plan Ahead

By planning ahead, you can avoid travel-related diabetes problems. If you notice signs of hypoglycemia, for example, you don't want to have to look for a rest stop when you're driving or wait for a flight attendant to bring you something to eat when you're flying. Keep snacks with you that could be used to prevent—or treat—low blood glucose, such as candy or small cans of juice.

Follow your meal plan as much as possible when you eat out. Carry a snack with you in case you have to wait to be served. If you're flying on one of those rare flights where any meals are served, request a diabetic meal in advance.

If You're Traveling with Insulin

Here are some tips for traveling with insulin:

- Carry your insulin in an insulated bag to keep it from freezing or getting too hot.
- Bring extra supplies of insulin in case of loss or breakage.
- Carry extra blood-glucose-monitoring supplies.
- Be sure to carry a letter from your doctor saying that you have diabetes and need insulin, syringes, and supplies for testing your blood glucose.
- Get a prescription for your insulin from your doctor in case you have to purchase some while you are away. A few states and several foreign countries require a prescription for insulin and syringes.

During Travel

The paramount rule of travel for a person with diabetes is this: Keep your diabetes supplies with you. If you're flying, keep your supplies in your carry-on luggage (never check them through). If you're driving, make sure they remain within reach. And wherever you go, don't forget to carry extra supplies—medication, insulin, and syringes. It may be hard to find them in unfamiliar places.

Carry your glucose monitor and supplies, and check your blood glucose often. If you're taking a long trip, test before you start out and then every two hours during the trip. Carry snacks to ward off hypoglycemia.

Bring your medicines in their original pharmacy containers with the printed label that identifies what they are and how they are to be taken. Don't count on buying more if you run out. The types of insulin and drugs sold outside the United States often differ markedly from those available at home, starting with their names.

Wear a medical alert bracelet or necklace that identifies you as a diabetic. Let your travel companion or trip leader know what to do if you show signs of hypoglycemia (see chapter 10).

People with diabetes should pay special attention to footwear and, when traveling, always wear comfortable, well-fitting shoes. This is particularly important, of course, if you're going to be walking a lot. Remember to check for blisters or other injuries to your feet (see chapter 11) to prevent more serious problems.

Try to maintain your normal schedule. If you usually test your blood glucose at noon and then eat lunch, for example, plan to do this on your trip as well. Traveling will very likely entail delays in, and changes to, your daily routine. Restaurant food will differ from what you eat at home. But if you know what to expect, you can plan to eat healthfully and manage your diabetes under unusual circumstances while sampling different cuisines.

Enjoy Your Trip

Having diabetes doesn't mean you must compromise on your choice of vacations. True, you'll face particular challenges if you're planning to climb Mount Everest or live in the wild for an extended period. For more conventional jaunts, however, you can go just about anywhere and do just about anything you like. All it takes is some advance planning, a consultation with your health care provider, and a little extra attention and self care.

APPENDIX D

Diabetes Emergencies

Some diabetes emergencies require urgent care. Here is a brief summary of common emergencies that people with diabetes may experience, along with some suggested basic action steps for how to deal with them.

Take Immediate Action

Get emergency help or call 911 immediately if you, a family member, or a friend with diabetes has any of these symptoms:

- Blood glucose is over 500 mg/dL.
- Urine has medium or large amounts of ketones.
- Low blood glucose does not return to normal after two treatments with 10 to 15 grams of fast-acting sugar. (See the table on page 123.)
- The person with diabetes cannot swallow or loses consciousness, and glucagon is not available.

Talk to your family, friends, and co-workers about what to do in case of a diabetic emergency. Being prepared and monitoring your blood glucose frequently will prevent most emergencies.

Hypoglycemia

Hypoglycemia means that you have too much insulin and not enough glucose in your blood. It may occur when you don't eat enough, when you wait too long to eat, when too much medication is in your body, or when you use glucose faster than usual. Sometimes exercise can cause hypoglycemia.

Symptoms

- Nervousness and shakiness
- Perspiration
- Dizziness or light-headedness
- Sleepiness
- Confusion
- Difficulty speaking
- Hunger
- Feeling anxious or weak

Home care

- Eat or drink 10 to 15 grams of a fast-acting sugar. (See the table on page 123.) Once blood glucose returns to normal, eat a snack if your next meal is more than 30 minutes away. If blood glucose is not normal within 15 to 20 minutes, eat another snack. If blood-glucose levels don't return to normal after the second snack, seek emergency care.

- If you can't swallow or if you pass out, someone should give you a glucagon shot. If glucagon is not available, the person caring for you can rub sugar or cake frosting on the inside of your mouth. Teach your family and co-workers how to do these things before an emergency occurs.

You or the person caring for you should get emergency care right away if:

- Low blood glucose doesn't return to normal after two treatments with a 10 to 15 grams of fast-acting sugar.

- You cannot swallow or you pass out and glucagon is not available.

Ketones in the Blood (Diabetic Ketoacidosis)

Ketones are dangerous chemicals that can collect in your blood. You can detect them with a urine test.

Symptoms

Symptoms occur slowly, over 12 to 24 hours, and may include:

- Extreme thirst, dry mouth, and/or fruity breath
- Feeling sleepy or tired
- Feeling sick to the stomach or throwing up
- Going to the bathroom more often than usual
- Fever and/or warm, dry skin
- Trouble breathing
- Pain in the lower stomach
- Lack of hunger

Home care

- Drink a glass of water every hour.
- Call your doctor if you find small amounts of ketones in your urine.
- If you find medium or large amounts of ketones in your urine, get emercency care right away.

Hyperglycemia

Hyperglycemia means you have too much glucose and not enough insulin in your blood. It may occur when you eat too much, when you do not take your insulin as directed, or if you skip your regular exercise.

Symptoms

- Extreme thirst and/or warm, dry skin
- Feeling sleepy
- More frequent urination than usual

Home care

- Follow your doctor's instructions. He or she may tell you to take an extra dose of insulin or medication when you experience hyperglycemia, or to exercise.

• Test your blood glucose often.

• If your blood glucose is over 240 mg/dL, check your urine for ketones.

Call your doctor if:

• Your blood glucose does not come down or you do not feel better two hours after starting home care.

• Ketones are present in your urine.

Hyperglycemic Hyperosmolar Nonketonic Syndrome (HHNS)

HHNS happens when an extremely high level of glucose in the blood causes severe dehydration. It usually takes several days—possibly even weeks—for HHNS to develop.

Symptoms

Symptoms occur slowly, over several days, and can include:

• Extreme thirst; dry mouth
• Blurred vision
• Hallucinations
• Feeling sleepy or confused
• Weakness on one side of the body
• High fever and/or warm, dry skin

Home care

When you are sick, drink a glass of water every hour and test your blood glucose more often. Even minor illnesses can raise your blood-glucose levels.

• Call your physician if your blood glucose is over 350 mg/dL.

• Get emergency help right away if your blood glucose is over 600 mg/dL.

Index

mixing, 64–65
oral, 166
patches, 74, 166
precautions when using, 68–69
pre-mixes, 59
pumps, 40, 73–74
rapid-acting, 58, 59
role of, 57
short-acting, 58
side effects of, 69–70
storing, 71
therapy, 57–74
times to take, 59–60
traveling with, 188
treatment, 39–40
 for type 2 diabetes, 78
 in type 1 diabetes, 8
 in type 2 diabetes, 6–7
types of, 58–59
Insurance, 183
Islet-cell transplants, 164–165

JDRF. See Juvenile Diabetes
 Research Foundation
Jefferson, Thomas, 36
Journal of the American Medical
 Association, 114
Juvenile Diabetes Research
 Foundation (JDRF), 171

Ketoacidosis. See Diabetic
 ketoacidosis
Ketones, 5, 8, 41, 184, 191–192
 testing for, 42
Ketosis, 5

Kidney problems, 14, 60,
 136–138
 diagnosing, 138
 transplants and, 164
 treating, 138

Labels, food, 92–93
Lancets, 48
 drawing blood with, 49
 new types of, 56
Lantus, 59
Laser photocoagulation, 142
Leg pain, 132
Lente, 58
Levemir, 59
Lifestyle, 151–162, 181–183
Limits, setting, 160
Lipid levels, 127
Lispro, 58
Long-term complications,
 125–149, 180–181
 preventing, 126
"Low fat," 93
Lubricants, 159

Magnesium, 22, 116–117
Marriage therapists, 33
Massage, 179
Maturity-onset diabetes in the
 young (MODY), 11
Mayo Clinic, 114
Meal planning, 21–22, 30, 36–37,
 81–97, 160, 174–176
 balancing meals in, 89
 for diabetes types, 81–82

Vaginal dryness, 157, 159

Vasocongestion, 157

Vision, blurry, 23

Vitrectomy, 142

Vodka, 97

Vomiting, 60

Warming up, 105

Weight, 19, 99

  control, 176–178

  losing, 24–25, 175

Weight Control Information
     Network (WIN), 178

WIN. See Weight Control
     Information Network

Wine, 97

Workout plans, 102–103. See also
     Exercise

Yeast infections, 157

Yoga, 177